HERPES

Anthrax

Campylobacteriosis

Cholera

Escherichia coli Infections

Gonorrhea

Hepatitis

Herpes

HIV/AIDS

Influenza

Lyme Disease

Mad Cow Disease (Bovine Spongiform Encephalopathy)

Malaria

Meningitis

Mononucleosis

Plague

Polio

SARS

Smallpox

Streptococcus (Group A)

Syphilis

Toxic Shock Syndrome

Tuberculosis

Typhoid Fever

West Nile Virus

DEADLY DISEASES AND EPIDEMICS

HERPES

Juliet V. Spencer

CONSULTING EDITOR
The Late I. Edward Alcamo
Distinguished Teaching Professor of Microbiology,
SUNY Farmingdale

FOREWORD BY
David Heymann
World Health Organization

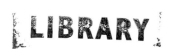

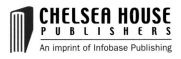

CHELSEA HOUSE
PUBLISHERS
An imprint of Infobase Publishing

Dedication
We dedicate the books in the DEADLY DISEASES AND EPIDEMICS series to Ed Alcamo, whose wit, charm, intelligence, and commitment to biology education were second to none.

Herpes

Chelsea House
An imprint of Infobase Publishing
132 West 31st Street
New York NY 10001

ISBN-10: 0-7910-8196-6
ISBN-13: 978-0-7910-8196-9

Library of Congress Cataloging-in-Publication Data
Spencer, Juliet V.
   Herpes/Juliet V. Spencer
      p. cm.—(Deadly diseases and epidemics)
   ISBN 0-7910-8196-6 (hc)
   1. Herpesvirus diseases. 2. Herpes genitalis. I. Title. II. Series.
   RC203.H45S665 2005
   616.95'18—dc22   2004029798

Chelsea House books are available at special discounts when purchased in bulk quantities for businesses, associations, institutions, or sales promotions. Please call our Special Sales Department in New York at (212) 967-8800 or (800) 322-8755.

You can find Chelsea House on the World Wide Web at
http://www.chelseahouse.com

Series design by Terry Mallon
Cover design by Keith Trego

Printed in China

Nordica 21C 10 9 8 7 6 5 4 3 2

This book is printed on acid-free paper.

All links and Web addresses were checked and verified to be correct at the time of publication. Because of the dynamic nature of the Web, some addresses and links may have changed since publication and may no longer be valid.

Table of Contents

Foreword

In the 1960s, many of the infectious diseases that had terrorized generations were tamed. After a century of advances, the leading killers of Americans both young and old were being prevented with new vaccines or cured with new medicines. The risk of death from pneumonia, tuberculosis (TB), meningitis, influenza, whooping cough, and diphtheria declined dramatically. New vaccines lifted the fear that summer would bring polio, and a global campaign was on the verge of eradicating smallpox worldwide. New pesticides like DDT cleared mosquitoes from homes and fields, thus reducing the incidence of malaria, which was present in the southern United States and which remains a leading killer of children worldwide. New technologies produced safe drinking water and removed the risk of cholera and other water-borne diseases. Science seemed unstoppable. Disease seemed destined to all but disappear.

But the euphoria of the 1960s has evaporated.

The microbes fought back. Those causing diseases like TB and malaria evolved resistance to cheap and effective drugs. The mosquito developed the ability to defuse pesticides. New diseases emerged, including AIDS, Legionnaires, and Lyme disease. And diseases which had not been seen in decades re-emerged, as the hantavirus did in the Navajo Nation in 1993. Technology itself actually created new health risks. The global transportation network, for example, meant that diseases like West Nile virus could spread beyond isolated regions and quickly become global threats. Even modern public health protections sometimes failed, as they did in 1993 in Milwaukee, Wisconsin, resulting in 400,000 cases of the digestive system illness cryptosporidiosis. And, more recently, the threat from smallpox, a disease believed to be completely eradicated, has returned along with other potential bioterrorism weapons such as anthrax.

The lesson is that the fight against infectious diseases will never end.

In our constant struggle against disease, we as individuals have a weapon that does not require vaccines or drugs, and that is the warehouse of knowledge. We learn from the history of science that "modern" beliefs can be wrong. In this series of books, for example, you will learn that diseases like syphilis were once thought to be caused by eating potatoes. The invention of the microscope set science on the right path. There are more positive lessons from history. For example, smallpox was eliminated by vaccinating everyone who had come in contact with an infected person. This "ring" approach to smallpox control is still the preferred method for confronting an outbreak, should the disease be intentionally reintroduced.

At the same time, we are constantly adding new drugs, new vaccines, and new information to the warehouse. Recently, the entire human genome was decoded. So too was the genome of the parasite that causes malaria. Perhaps by looking at the microbe and the victim through the lens of genetics we will be able to discover new ways to fight malaria, which remains the leading killer of children in many countries.

Because of advances in our understanding of such diseases as AIDS, entire new classes of anti-retroviral drugs have been developed. But resistance to all these drugs has already been detected, so we know that AIDS drug development must continue.

Education, experimentation, and the discoveries that grow out of them are the best tools to protect health. Opening this book may put you on the path of discovery. I hope so, because new vaccines, new antibiotics, new technologies, and, most importantly, new scientists are needed now more than ever if we are to remain on the winning side of this struggle against microbes.

David Heymann
Executive Director
Communicable Diseases Section
World Health Organization
Geneva, Switzerland

1

A Painful Discovery

Teresa was starting to get nervous. The elation she had felt after the magical evening of the prom was starting wear off, and in its place was an increasingly painful itchiness and a cluster of small blisters in her groin region. Last Friday had been Prom Night, and Teresa had attended with Sean, her boyfriend of the past five months. Sean had been so dashing and handsome in his black tuxedo, with a red cummerbund to match her red taffeta dress. The corsage he had presented her with contained red and white rosebuds with delicate baby's breath. They had danced all night, and then attended a party at their friend Steven Nelson's house. Steven's parents were out of town, and Teresa and Sean had sneaked upstairs to an empty bedroom. With the lights down low, amid warm memories of the romantic evening, Teresa had been more than willing when Sean asked if she wanted to go "all the way." Even though the condom broke when he was putting it on, Teresa told Sean it was okay to continue. Her mother had taken her to the doctor to start a prescription for birth control pills several months ago, so there was no chance that Teresa would get pregnant.

As Teresa looked back on the evening, she realized that having sex without a condom probably wasn't such a great idea after all. The birth control pills would prevent her from getting pregnant, but they wouldn't protect her from getting a disease like AIDS. It was hard to imagine that Sean might have HIV, the virus that causes AIDS, but at the same time, she was itchy and achy and something was very definitely wrong. With one more glance at the dried corsage she was so carefully trying to preserve, Teresa fought back tears as she went downstairs to talk to her mother.

After visiting her family doctor, Teresa was relieved to learn that she probably did not have HIV, although that would have to be confirmed

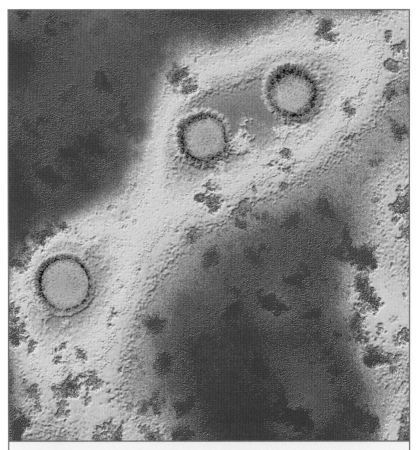

Figure 1.1 Herpes simplex virus (HSV) is the agent that causes both cold sores and genital herpes. This image, taken with a transmission electron microscope, shows virus particles inside an infected cell magnified 200,000 times.

by a blood test in about six months. Rather, the doctor had diagnosed **genital herpes**. Laboratory tests would later confirm his diagnosis, but in the meantime, the doctor had given Teresa a prescription for medication to help ease her symptoms. The painful blisters, the doctor had explained, were most likely caused by the **herpes simplex virus** (**HSV**) (Figure 1.1). The blisters would go away, but the virus that caused them would not. Teresa would remain infected for life, and would probably experience outbreaks of the blisters periodically. Although people carrying HSV can live perfectly normal lives, Teresa would need to monitor the status of her outbreaks to avoid passing the virus on to future sexual partners.

Stories like Teresa's are not uncommon today. Sexually transmitted diseases such as herpes are on the rise, and the use of oral contraceptives offers no protection from the **pathogens** that cause them. The herpes simplex virus belongs to a family of viruses known as the *Herpesviridae*. The name *herpes* comes from the Greek word meaning "to creep," which is a reference to the spreading skin lesions found in affected people. Herpes viruses are widespread in the population. Overall, about 50% of the general population is infected with a herpes virus, but in lower socioeconomic groups the infection rate can be much higher, up to 80 to 90%, due to poor hygiene, lack of health education, or inadequate health care. There are eight human herpes viruses (see Table 1.1), all of which can cause illnesses that are usually mild or even **asymptomatic**, although occasionally they are associated with severely life-threatening infections. Varicella zoster virus is well known as the cause of chicken pox, a common childhood infection, and also shingles, a painful rash that affects mainly the elderly. Epstein-Barr virus is contracted by many people at a young age with little apparent disease, but in teens and young adults it can cause mononucleosis, an illness characterized by fever, fatigue, sore throat, and swollen lymph glands that can last for several months. HSV can cause **oral herpes**, the skin lesions commonly called fever blisters or cold sores on the face near the mouth (Figure 1.2), as well as genital herpes.

There are actually two types of herpes simplex viruses: HSV-1 and HSV-2. Oral herpes is usually caused by HSV-1, and the majority of genital herpes cases are caused by HSV-2. Physicians used to say that above the belt, the infection was due to HSV-1; below the belt, HSV-2. However, both type-1 and

Table 1.1 **Human Herpes Viruses**

HERPES VIRUS	COMMON NAME	CLINICAL SYNDROMES
HHV-1	Herpes simplex virus type 1 (HSV-1)	Fever blisters
HHV-2	Herpes simplex virus type 2 (HSV-2)	Genital herpes
HHV-3	Varicella zoster virus	Chicken pox, shingles
HHV-4	Epstein-Barr virus	Mononucleosis, Burkitt's lymphoma
HHV-5	Cytomegalovirus	Neonatal birth defects
HHV-6	Human herpes virus 6	Roseola infantum
HHV-7	Human herpes virus 7	Roseola infantum
HHV-8	Kaposi's sarcoma–associated herpes virus	Kaposi's sarcoma

type-2 can occur in the genitals, facial region, or both. If a person with HSV-1 oral herpes performs oral sex, it is possible for the partner to contract genital herpes caused by HSV-1 infection. Likewise, a person could develop HSV-2 oral fever blisters as a result of oral sexual contact with HSV-2 infected

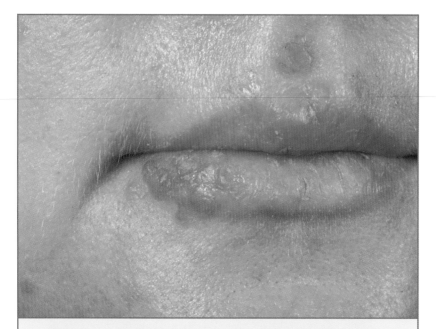

Figure 1.2 Herpes simplex viruses can infect the skin in the face and mouth region, resulting in small, sometimes painful, fluid-filled blisters (seen here). The fluid inside the fever blisters is filled with infectious virus, and can be passed on to others through kissing or other direct contact. Once the blisters dry out and scab over, transmission of the virus is less likely.

genitals. The herpes virus is transmitted by direct skin-to-skin contact. This occurs when a contagious area (such as a blister) comes into contact with a mucous membrane, such as the lining of the mouth or genitals. Most skin on the body is too thick for the virus to go through, although having tiny breaks in the skin, as from a cut, greatly increases the chance of virus infection. There are no documented cases of a person getting herpes from an inanimate object, such as a toilet seat, bathtub, or towel. Herpes is a fragile virus and does not survive for very long on inanimate objects and surfaces.

What are the symptoms of a genital herpes infection? In many cases, the infection is asymptomatic, meaning that there are no obvious signs or symptoms. Alternatively, as was the case with Teresa, infection may be evident several days after exposure to the virus. When present, the symptoms generally include small sores, blisters, bumps, or a rash combined with itching, burning, or tingling in the genital area. The person may also develop flu-like symptoms, such as headache, fever, and swollen glands. The symptoms may last for several weeks, but on average they last for only 2 to 10 days. The severity of the symptoms varies greatly from person to person, as does the number of outbreaks. During an outbreak, the individual is contagious and can infect others. It is important to realize that even individuals without obvious symptoms can be contagious.

After the initial or **primary infection**, the herpes simplex virus can establish **latency**, a period of dormancy that is common to all herpes viruses. During latent periods, the person is not infectious, but the virus is lying in wait for its next opportunity to appear. Most infected individuals will probably experience an average of four to five genital herpes

(continued on page 16)

WHAT IS A VIRUS?

Prior to the late 19th century, it was not understood that infectious microorganisms (living things so small that they can only be seen through a microscope) could cause human disease. The work of scientists at the end of the 19th century established the germ theory of disease, the concept that infectious diseases are caused by microorganisms. As the germ theory took hold in the medical community, researchers began to identify the agents that caused human diseases. Robert Koch established a method by which an organism could be isolated from a sick animal or person, grown in a pure culture, and then used to infect a healthy individual, who later developed the same disease and carried the same organism. These steps, which came to be known as Koch's postulates, were first used to identify the bacterium that caused anthrax in cattle, *Bacillus anthracis*, and later the bacterium that caused tuberculosis in humans, *Mycobacterium tuberculosis*.

Still, researchers were unable to cultivate the causative agent for some diseases. For example, Louis Pasteur had difficulty isolating the microorganism that caused rabies. Pasteur was able to reproduce the disease in dogs and rabbits injected with brain tissue from an infected animal, and this led him to suggest that the agent of the disease was too small to be seen. The science of **virology** was born when one of Pasteur's colleagues, Charles Chamberland, developed a porcelain bacterial filter. (**Virologists** are scientists who study viruses and their structure, replication, and interactions with host cells.) Dmitri Ivanowski used Chamberland's filter to study tobacco mosaic disease, and he showed that leaf extracts from infected plants could cause disease in healthy plants even after filtration to remove bacteria. It soon became clear that these filterable organisms were different from bacteria. These agents—now known as viruses—were soon identified as the cause of foot-and-mouth disease of cattle, yellow fever in humans, and many other diseases.

A **virus** is basically a microscopic packet of genetic material surrounded by a protein coat, or **capsid** (Figure 1.3). One reason that viruses could not be cultivated on a growth medium in the same way that bacteria had been isolated is that viruses must be grown in cells, such as in the tissues of a host organism or in animal cells in *in vitro* systems. (*In vitro* literally means "in glass" and refers to biological processes occurring outside of a living organism; in this case, viral infection of cells grown in a laboratory culture dish.) When a virus infects a host cell, it directs the cell's metabolic machinery to make more viruses. The outcome of virus infection varies depending on the virus; in some cases, there is little impact on the cell, and in other cases, the cell dies. Viruses can attack almost any cellular organism, including plants, animals, and even bacteria. Even today there is some debate among scientists as to whether viruses should be classified as living organisms. Viruses have the ability to reproduce, evolve, and adapt to changing environmental conditions, and they contain many of the same **enzymes**, nucleic acids, carbohydrates, and lipids found in living cells. On the other hand, viruses are not cells, and they lack the ability to carry out metabolism or reproduction without the aid of a living cell.

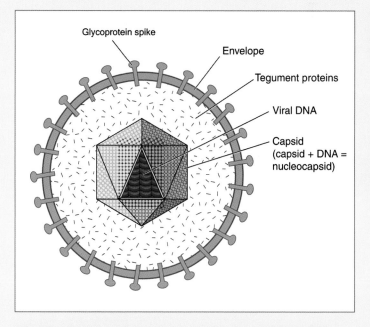

Glycoprotein spike

Envelope

Tegument proteins

Viral DNA

Capsid
(capsid + DNA =
nucleocapsid)

Figure 1.3 Illustrated here is a herpes virus particle. The icosahedral (20-sided) capsid houses the viral DNA and is surrounded by a mass of **tegument** proteins. The entire particle is enclosed in a membrane envelope, which contains **glycoprotein spikes** protruding from the surface. These glycoprotein spikes attach to receptors on host cells, allowing the virus to adhere to and penetrate the cell.

(continued from page 13)

outbreaks a year. Generally, the first outbreak is the most extreme, and recurrent outbreaks tend to lessen in frequency and severity over time. Outbreaks may be triggered by illness, poor diet, stress, or a variety of other factors. The frequency of outbreaks can be decreased through nutrition, exercise, getting enough sleep, and effective stress management. Unfortunately, Teresa, and many others like her, will have to deal with recurrent outbreaks from HSV-2 for the rest of her life. It is estimated that over 25% of the adult population is currently infected with HSV-2.

This book aims to educate the reader about the nature of herpes and its treatment. Chapter 2 discusses the **epidemiology**, or frequency and distribution, of genital herpes and other sexually transmitted diseases. The structure of the virus is discussed in Chapter 3, and its replication cycle is described in Chapter 4. In Chapter 5, we will look at virus latency, an unusual aspect of virus infection that is common to all herpes viruses. Chapter 6 discusses other clinical syndromes that can result from herpes simplex infections, and Chapter 7 outlines the diagnosis and treatment of the infections. Chapter 8 presents an overview of the status of prevention and control methods to stop the spread of HSV, and Chapter 9 describes what the future may hold for the virus and those who are infected.

2

Epidemiology of Sexually Transmitted Diseases

In Chapter 1, we met Teresa, a sexually active teen who was responsible enough to realize that sexual intercourse could result in pregnancy. Although she had taken steps to prevent pregnancy by taking birth control pills, Teresa could still have been exposed to a number of **sexually transmitted diseases** (**STDs**) in addition to herpes. In this chapter, we look at the factors that contribute to the rapid spread of sexually transmitted diseases, with specific information about how genital herpes is contracted and the current statistics on the HSV epidemic. Some of the most frequently asked questions about STDs and genital herpes will be answered here.

WHAT IS AN STD?

Sexually transmitted diseases (STDs) are infectious diseases that are spread though sexual activity, such as vaginal intercourse, anal intercourse, and oral-genital or oral-anal contact. Sexually transmitted diseases have also been called venereal diseases, a name derived from Venus, the Roman goddess of love, beauty, and fertility. The most common STDs are chlamydia, gonorrhea, syphilis, genital warts, and genital herpes (Table 2.1). Human immunodeficiency virus (HIV), the virus that causes AIDS, can also be classified as an STD.

WHAT FACTORS CONTRIBUTE TO THE SPREAD OF STDS?

In the United States today, more than 65 million people are infected with some type of incurable STD (about 75% of these cases are genital herpes versus 1.4% for HIV), and it is estimated that there are 15 million

Table 2.1 Sexually Transmitted Diseases

DISEASE	INFECTIOUS AGENT	INCIDENCE*	CURABLE	TREATMENT
Chlamydia	Chlamydia trachomatis	3 million	Yes	Doxycycline, erythromycin
Gonorrhea	Neisseria gonorrhoeae	650,000	Yes	Ciprofloxacin
Syphilis	Treponema pallidum	34,000	Yes	Penicillin
Genital herpes	Herpes simplex virus (HSV)	1 million	No	Acyclovir, valacyclovir
Condyloma acuminata (genital warts)	Human papillomavirus (HPV)	5.5 million	No	None
AIDS	Human immuno-deficiency virus (HIV)	40,000	No	Retrovir®, indinavir (17 drugs available)

* Incidence refers to the number of new cases reported per year. Local health department officials require that physicians report certain diseases for public health records and epidemiological tracking purposes. Chlamydia, gonorrhea, syphilis, and AIDS are all reportable diseases by law. In contrast, diagnoses of genital herpes and genital warts are not required to be reported to public health officials.

new STD cases each year. Most adults in the United States contract at least one STD before the age of 35.

Just prior to World War II (1939–1945), there was a dramatic increase in the incidence of STDs, particularly syphilis and gonorrhea. In the 1940s, a public health campaign was launched to warn soldiers of the dangers of casual sex (Figure 2.1). Fortunately, the discovery of antibiotics such as penicillin and streptomycin allowed for effective treatment of these bacterial diseases, and until the 1970s, many physicians believed that STDs would soon be eliminated through the use of antibiotics. Not only did STDs fail to disappear, but the problem has actually worsened. Several factors have contributed to the rise of STDs since the 1970s: the emergence of antibiotic-resistant strains, the widespread use of oral contraceptives, and the emergence of new pathogens.

ANTIBIOTIC RESISTANCE

The discovery of penicillin was a major step forward in controlling gonorrhea, one of the first identified STDs. Incidence of gonorrhea had soared during the 1940s, but the previously untreatable illness was now easily cured with a simple injection of penicillin. Over time, however, the microorganism that causes gonorrhea, *Neisseria gonorrhoeae*, has developed resistance to this powerful antibiotic. Bacteria develop antibiotic resistance through chromosomal mutations or by acquiring an extra piece of genetic material called a **plasmid**, which is a common event for bacteria. Plasmids that convey resistance to penicillin generally encode a gene for **beta-lactamase**, an enzyme that destroys penicillin. Although other drugs are currently available to treat gonorrhea, they are much more expensive than penicillin, and this has caused a major problem for publicly funded health clinics. In addition, it is not known how long these drugs will remain effective, since drug-resistant strains continue to emerge.

Despite concerns over antibiotic resistance, it remains relatively easy to treat STDs caused by bacterial infections, especially

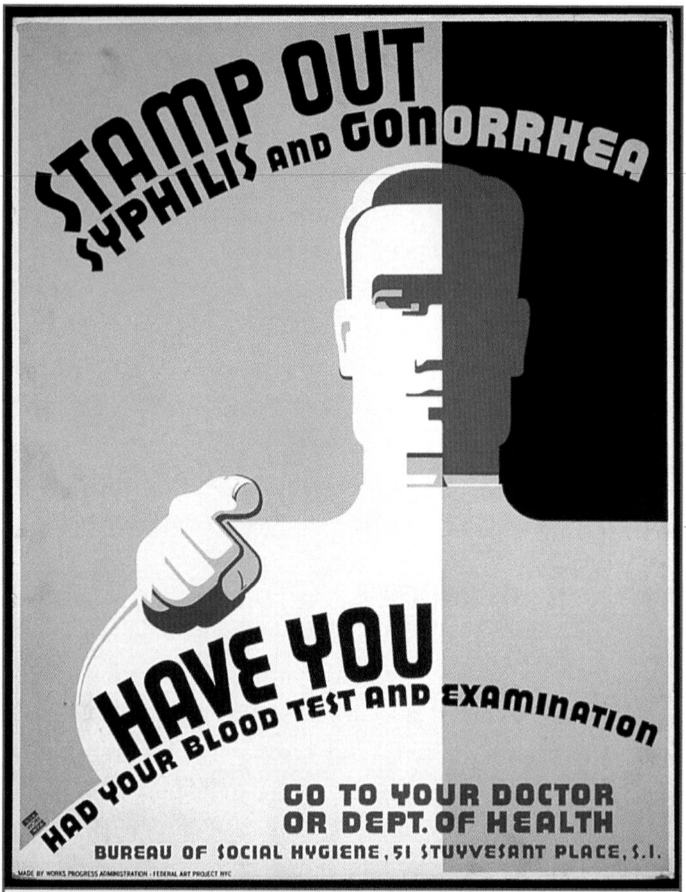

Figure 2.1 Public health posters, such as the one shown here, were designed in the 1940s to warn both soldiers and the general public of the dangers of sexually transmitted disease. Films, lectures, pamphlets, and demonstrations were also used by public health educators, but posters were particularly well suited for campaigns designed to appeal to a broad range of servicemen and the general public.

the more prevalent diseases such as syphilis, gonorrhea, and chlamydia. Viral infections, on the other hand, are not treatable with antibiotics, and effective medications for genital herpes, human papillomavirus, and HIV remain to be discovered.

BIRTH CONTROL PILLS

The introduction of birth control pills in the early 1960s enabled women to control their own fertility. Birth control pills are synthetic hormones that mimic the way that the real hormones estrogen and progestin work in a women's body. The pill prevents ovulation; a woman on the pill releases no new eggs, since her body is tricked into believing she is already pregnant. By using oral contraception, women could put off motherhood to pursue education and a career, without having to abstain from sex. The widespread use of birth control pills, together with the rise of the feminist movement, social activism, and individualistic thinking, contributed to the sexual freedom of the late 1960s and 1970s. For the first time, women could have intercourse without the worry of getting pregnant. Unfortunately, the protection offered by the birth control pill did not (and still does not) extend to sexually transmitted diseases. The introduction of birth control pills coincided with the beginning of an upswing in the number of STDs reported annually. It is essential for women who take the pill to understand that they are still at risk of contracting STDs unless their partner has tested negative or uses a condom.

NEW PATHOGENS

It is difficult to find anyone today who has not heard of human immunodeficiency virus (HIV), the virus that causes AIDS. However, this lethal virus was discovered only in the early 1980s. HIV is a retrovirus that inserts its genetic material into the host's genetic material, or deoxyribonucleic acid (DNA), a characteristic that makes it very difficult to eliminate from the body. In addition, the initial infection is usually very mild, with flu-like symptoms. After that initial exposure, individuals may go for years without experiencing any symptoms of disease and believe that they are disease-free. During this period, however, the individuals are still contagious and capable of infecting sexual partners with HIV. There is no cure for HIV, and in many patients the virus infection progresses to the point that it causes AIDS, a disease in which the immune system is weakened and unable to fight a number of serious and fatal infections. Since 1981, more than 20 million people worldwide have died from AIDS. Perhaps because of its deadly toll, the publicity surrounding this incurable STD has actually served to raise awareness of other STDs. Since the early 1990s, there has been a slight downward trend for many STDs, an observation that has been correlated with increased condom use for prevention of HIV infection. In the United States, there are currently around 950,000 known HIV-positive individuals, with about 40,000 new cases diagnosed each year. One particularly dangerous trend is the recent observation by doctors and scientists that people with genital herpes are at increased risk of contracting HIV, due to the presence of open blisters or sores that allow HIV direct access to the bloodstream.

HOW WIDESPREAD IS GENITAL HERPES?

More than one in five Americans (over 45 million people in the United States) are infected with genital herpes. Since the late 1970s, the number of Americans with genital herpes infections increased by 30%, with the largest increases seen in adolescents in the 12- to 19-year-old age group. Approximately 1 million additional cases are reported each year. Ironically, in a national survey, fewer than 10% of those who tested positive for genital herpes knew they were infected, suggesting that the current estimate of 45 million HSV-2 positive adults may be significantly lower than the actual number. Some health officials believe the number is closer to 60 million and still growing. Because genital herpes is incurable, the total number of infected persons in the population will likely continue to rise until an effective vaccine strategy is developed.

HOW DO PEOPLE GET GENITAL HERPES?

HSV is spread by direct contact, or skin-to-skin transfer. Infectious virus is present in the blisters or sores that can occur in the affected area. When the blisters or the liquid from them comes into contact with a susceptible area of another person's body, that person can become infected, too. The most susceptible areas are the **mucous membranes** that cover all of the body's interior surfaces, such as the mouth and digestive tract as well as the genitourinary system (Figure 2.2). Although our skin is a relatively thick and impermeable covering of the body's exterior surfaces, mucous membranes are much thinner and provide less of a protective barrier from foreign invaders. Transmission is more common from men to women, possibly because the exposed membrane surface of the vagina is greater than that of the penis. Vaginal intercourse, anal intercourse, and oral sex are all ways that HSV can be transmitted from one person to another. In addition to gaining entry at the mucous membranes, the herpes virus can also enter the body through small breaks in

RETROVIRUSES

Retroviruses are viruses that use RNA (ribonucleic acid) as their genetic material rather than DNA. There are many RNA viruses, but retroviruses replicate (multiply) in a very distinct fashion. The term *retro* is derived from the Latin for "backward" and it refers to an unusual step in the replication cycle of these viruses. Whereas most organisms use DNA to make RNA (and most RNA viruses use only RNA), retroviruses use the reverse process to make DNA. This unique reaction requires an enzyme called reverse transcriptase, which is present in the retrovirus. After the RNA genome is reverse-transcribed into a DNA copy, known as a provirus, the provirus integrates into the host genome. This means that the DNA sequence inserts itself into the cell's DNA and becomes a permanent part of the cell. The provirus is replicated along with host cell DNA so that every time the cell divides, the resulting daughter cells always contain the provirus. When the viral genes are expressed, the cell produces new infectious retroviruses.

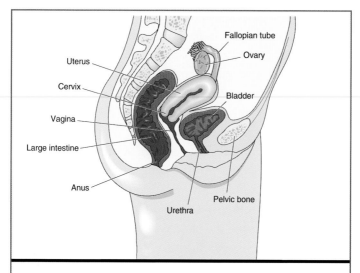

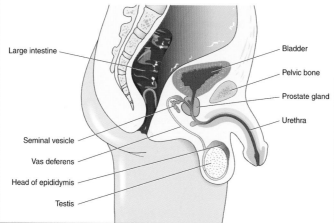

Figure 2.2 Illustrated here is the genitourinary system of a female (top) and male (bottom). In the female anatomy, the reproductive system and urinary system are separate, which means there is additional mucous membrane surface. The membranes on the lining of the urethra, vagina, and anus are all potential sites for infection with HSV. Because most of these surfaces are internal, a woman may be infected and still lack any visible lesions. The male anatomy is designed differently, with the urethra carrying both urine and sperm, but this mucous membrane is less exposed.

the skin. Because of the intimate contact that accompanies sexual intercourse, virtually any area covered by a pair of shorts represents a possible site of genital herpes infection.

One of the biggest factors contributing to the rapid spread of genital herpes is the fact that infectious virus can still be released, or shed, even when there are no visible sores or blisters on the skin. This means that people who don't know they are infected or even those who believe they aren't currently contagious can still infect their sexual partners. The more partners an infected person has, the faster the spread of the disease (Figure 2.3) Asymptomatic transmission is the rule for genital herpes, not the exception. In this case, what you can't see *can* hurt you!

Another means of transmission of herpes is from mother to child during pregnancy. Most commonly, a mother who has an outbreak of genital herpes at the time of delivery can infect the newborn child as it passes through the birth canal. It is also possible for the virus to infect the fetus while still in the uterus, possibly through a small break in the amniotic membrane or if the membrane ruptures prematurely. In the event of neonatal herpes, the newborn generally develops lesions 5 to 10 days after birth. **Perinatal** transmission can be avoided by delivering the baby via caesarean section.

HOW CAN GENITAL HERPES AND OTHER STDS BE AVOIDED?

The greatest risk factors for contracting genital herpes and other STDs are having intercourse without a condom and having multiple sex partners. With more than one in five adults currently infected, exposure to HSV for most sexually active people is virtually guaranteed. Thus, the best way to avoid transmission of STDs, including genital herpes, is to abstain from sexual contact. Alternatively, a long-term mutually monogamous relationship with a partner who has tested negative is another safe option.

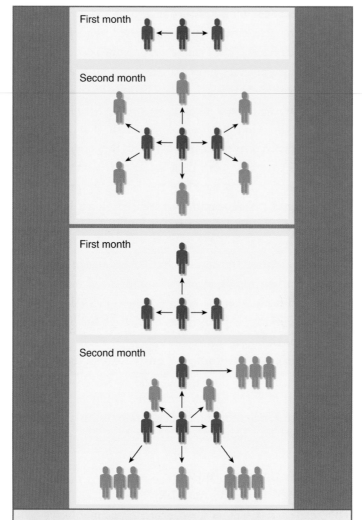

Figure 2.3 The role of multiple partners in the spread of sexually transmitted disease is illustrated here. If one person has unprotected sex with two partners in a month, the initially infected person can spread STDs to his or her partners. By the second month, if the first infected individual and the newly infected partners all continue to engage in unprotected sex with two new partners each, a total of nine people will be infected. If each person has three partners a month instead of two, the infection rate rises dramatically.

Although condoms have proven effective at preventing the transmission of some STDs, they are not 100% effective at preventing transmission of genital herpes, since blisters may occur in areas not covered by the condom, such as the inner thighs or around the anus. Individuals with herpes should refrain from sexual activity with an uninfected partner when lesions or other symptoms of herpes are present. However, since a person without any symptoms can still infect his or her sex partners, it is important to talk about your condition with your partner prior to having sexual relations. Many people find the topic uncomfortable and prefer to avoid the subject, but this evasion just contributes to the spread of STDs. An infected person must advise new sex partners of his or her status and the risk of becoming infected. Individuals who are not infected need to ask new sex partners directly whether they have been tested for genital herpes and other STDs.

Along the same lines, persons who develop genital lesions due to HSV-2 should recognize that unless they have recently tested negative, their infection could represent the reactivation of a previously unknown infection rather than a new infection traceable to a recent sexual partner. Relationships can be complicated enough without having suspicions and accusations get in the way.

While genital herpes (usually caused by HSV-2) is spread through sexual contact, it should be noted that many people are exposed to HSV-1 through more casual contact. The cold sores that can appear on lips or just inside the mouth are essentially the same as genital lesions in that they are full of infectious virus. Many children become infected with HSV-1 early in life when they are kissed by relatives with a cold sore. Just like genital herpes, cold sores can periodically reappear, usually as a result of stress, lack of sleep, poor diet, or a severe sunburn. People who are infected with HSV-1 can still become infected with HSV-2, and vice versa.

3

Nature's Design: Virus Structure

Viruses are always described as being small, tiny, or even microscopic. If you could actually see a herpes virus, what would it look like? And how small is it really? In this chapter, we describe the virus particle and the sophisticated equipment that would be needed to actually visualize it. Just to give you an idea of the size of the virus, if the period at the end of this sentence were a droplet of virus, you could fit more than 10,000 herpes viruses side by side across it. And HSV is one of the larger viruses! For a smaller virus like the poliovirus, you could fit more than 100,000 virus particles in that space.

One of the major ways viruses are categorized is by shape, and viruses in the *Herpesviridae* family share the same basic **morphology**, or structure. The complete genetic material, or **genome**, of these viruses consists of a single deoxyribonucleic acid (DNA) molecule enclosed in a protein capsid arranged in the shape of an icosahedron, a 20-sided figure. The capsid is covered by a dense protein layer called the tegument, and the entire particle is surrounded by an outer envelope containing numerous glycoprotein spikes. In this chapter, we will describe the molecular detail of each part of the virus particle: the genome, the capsid, the tegument, and the envelope (Figure 3.1).

THE GENOME

The Human Genome Project, whose goal was to identify all the genes in human DNA, was successfully completed in 2003. By identifying all the genes, researchers can learn more about which genes play a role in diseases such as diabetes, cancer, and cardiovascular disease, and also learn

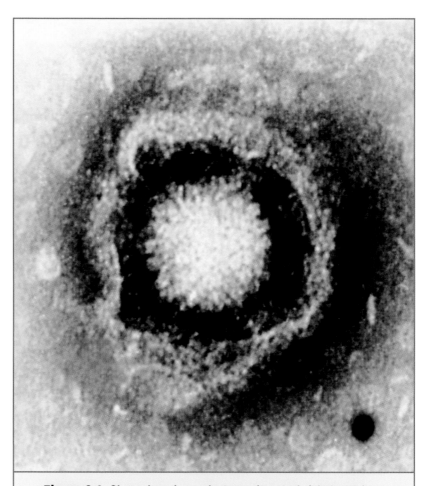

Figure 3.1 Shown here is an electron micrograph (photograph taken through a microscope) of the herpes simplex virus. The membrane envelope surrounding the particle is highly variable in shape. Capsid subunits, called capsomers, are clearly visible on the icosahedral shell. The capsid contains 162 capsomers, all of which are composed of the major capsid protein, encoded by the UL19 gene.

which genetic markers might make an individual more susceptible to those diseases. Once completed, all 3 billion base pairs of the human genome had been sequenced! By way of comparison, the genome of the herpes simplex virus consists

(continued on page 32)

THE CENTRAL DOGMA OF BIOLOGY

Most organisms store their genetic information in the form of DNA. This means that the sequence of the DNA molecules, or the organism's genome, contains all the instructions for every aspect of the organism. Like a molecular blueprint, our DNA contains information about our hair color, our height, and many other features. The information is encrypted in a DNA sequence, which consists of various combinations of the four nucleotide subunits of DNA: adenine, cytosine, guanine, and thymine (Figure 3.2). Hundreds or thousands of these bases in a row make up a gene, and these genes encode proteins that perform various functions in our bodies, from metabolizing sugar to making our bones strong.

However, since the genetic information in the DNA is so valuable and central to our functioning as humans, it is not accessed every time a new protein needs to be made. Rather, a copy of the desired gene is transcribed into a single-stranded molecule of ribonucleic acid (RNA), termed a *messenger RNA* (*mRNA*). **Transcription** is the process of producing an mRNA copy of a gene, and that mRNA copy is synthesized into protein through the process of **translation**. A single mRNA molecule can be used to make many copies of a protein. The flow of information from DNA to RNA to protein is known as the **central dogma of biology**. Viruses can take advantage of this process in that even with a relatively small genome, they can still produce many copies of the same protein for certain tasks, such as building a capsid shell.

For many years, scientists assumed that all organisms followed the central dogma, but we now know that certain viruses can use RNA as their main form of genetic storage and still have a DNA intermediate. **Retroviruses**, such as HIV, actually begin with RNA and make a DNA copy of their RNA genome, insert that viral DNA into the host's genome, and then proceed to make mRNA and protein in the host cell.

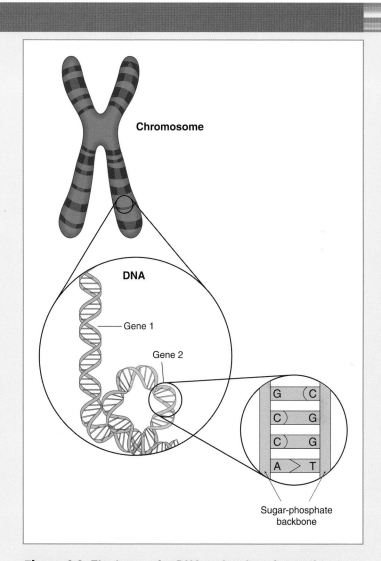

Figure 3.2 The bases of a DNA molecule pair together almost like the rungs of a ladder between two strands of sugar-phosphate backbone. The long DNA molecule is twisted into the shape of a double helix, and then further condensed with the aid of proteins into chromatin, the material that makes up human chromosomes.

(*continued from page 29*)

of a single linear DNA chromosome that is about 155,000 base pairs in length. If this DNA molecule were stretched out end to end, it would be 0.05 mm in length, which is about 250 times longer than the diameter of the entire virus particle. The HSV genome is composed of two segments of a unique DNA sequence that are flanked on either side by inverted repeat sequences. The two unique regions are called the Unique Long (UL) and Unique Short (US) segments, and they have the ability to invert relative to one another, resulting in four possible arrangements of the viral genetic material. The viral genes are designated in numerical order based on their location in the genome, and they are given the prefix UL, US, RL, or RS to denote genes in the UL and US components or repeat (R) sequences. For example, UL19 is the gene encoding the major capsid protein, which makes up the majority of the HSV capsid structure. The HSV-1 genome contains a total of 80 genes that encode 80 distinct proteins, while the HSV-2 has a total of 74 genes encoding 74 distinct proteins.

HSV genes are grouped into three categories depending upon their function. The three categories are: (1) regulation of viral gene expression, (2) DNA replication and associated functions, and (3) structure and assembly of the virus particle. One example of a regulatory component is the gene that encodes for the tegument protein UL41. UL41 is also known as *vhs*, or virus host shut-off, and this protein functions to prepare the host cell for virus replication by blocking its cellular DNA replication and protein synthesis.

Virus replication genes include a virally encoded DNA **polymerase** and other enzymes involved in nucleic acid metabolism and replication. Because the virus provides many of its own enzymes, HSV replication is not entirely dependent on the cell to provide replication enzymes. Whereas many viruses can only replicate in actively dividing cells—those that have replication enzymes readily available—HSV is cell-cycle independent. This means that HSV can replicate even in host cells that are not actively dividing, such as neurons (nerve cells, like those in the brain). This feature plays a key role in the ability of the virus to establish latency in neurons. Virus replication is described in greater detail in Chapter 4, and latency is discussed in Chapter 5.

During virus infection, the last genes to be transcribed are those that encode structural proteins that are involved in assembly of new virus particles. *Virion* is a term used to describe the complete virus particle, and about half of all the virally encoded proteins are either present in the virion or are required for virus assembly. Proteins present in the virion include glycoproteins found in the virus membrane, tegument proteins, and capsid proteins. In addition, several viral proteins are expressed in the host cell to aid with capsid assembly and packaging the viral genome into newly formed capsids, but these proteins are not found in the infectious virus particle.

THE CAPSID

Almost all virus capsids have one of two basic shapes (Figure 3.3). They are either helical, having a spiral configuration sort of like a phone cord, or icosahedral, having 20 triangular faces in a symmetrical sphere-like shape. What both of these shapes have in common is that they can be easily be made out of identical repeating subunits. Since the viral genome is relatively small (155,000 base pairs for HSV versus 3 billion base pairs for the human genome), it is beneficial for the virus to have just a few genes encoding proteins for the capsid and to use the host cell to make lots and lots of copies of those proteins. For HSV, there are four proteins present in the capsid, encoded by four viral genes. However, each virus capsid that is produced requires many copies of each protein; for example, 960 copies of the major capsid protein, encoded by the UL19 gene, are required to build just one capsid. In this way, hundreds of copies of each capsid protein can be produced by the host

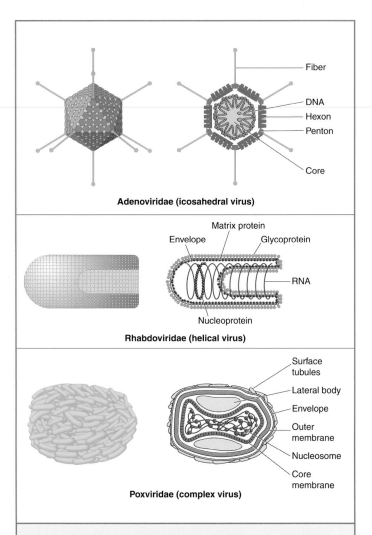

Fiber

DNA
Hexon
Penton

Core

Adenoviridae (icosahedral virus)

Matrix protein
Envelope   Glycoprotein

RNA

Nucleoprotein
Rhabdoviridae (helical virus)

Surface tubules
Lateral body
Envelope
Outer membrane
Nucleosome
Core membrane

Poxviridae (complex virus)

Figure 3.3 Three different virus structures are illustrated here. The icosahedral capsid is very common for virus particles; the herpes simplex virus and adenovirus (top) both use this 20-sided geometric shape to house their large genomes. The helical nucleocapsid (center) is common among RNA viruses like rabies (rhabdovirus) and influenza. There are very few viruses that have neither an icosahedral nor a helical capsid; poxvirus (bottom), the causative agent of smallpox, is one example of a complex capsid shape.

cell and assembled into the capsid, but only a small bit of the genome is devoted to encoding capsid proteins.

The major features of the capsid are 162 capsomers, or capsid subunits that protrude from the capsid floor. Of these capsomers, 150 are hexons, exhibiting six-fold symmetry, and 12 are pentons, exhibiting five-fold symmetry. Hexons are found on the faces and edges of the capsid, while pentons are found at each of the 12 vertices. The major capsid protein is the structural subunit of both hexons and pentons. Minor capsid proteins called UL18 and UL38 form trigonal nodules called triplexes that are located in the valleys between capsomers, connecting the capsomers in groups of three. An additional minor capsid protein, UL35, is found at the outer tips of the capsomers.

The HSV capsid is an icosahedral shell composed primarily of four proteins, although assembly of the capsid particle requires the aid of additional proteins. These **scaffolding**

(continued on page 38)

METHODS IN VIROLOGY: ELECTRON MICROSCOPY

If viruses are so tiny, how is it possible for scientists to describe what they look like? **Microscopy** is the use of light or electrons to magnify objects. In 1673, Antoni van Leeuwenhoek developed one of the first microscopes. His simple microscope was capable of magnifying objects 300 times, enabling him to observe small organisms in pond water. Simple microscopes were later replaced by compound microscopes, which use a series of lenses for magnification. Compound microscopes are found in most biology laboratories, and they consist of an eyepiece, or ocular lens, as well as an objective lens, with the total magnification being the product of the strength of each lens (i.e., a 10X eyepiece x 10X objective = 100X total magnification). Many compound microscopes have several different objective lenses mounted on a rotating nosepiece, which enable the viewer to achieve a total magnification ranging from 40X up to 2,000X. However, even a top-notch compound microscope cannot achieve magnification much greater than 2,000X. This is due to limitations in resolution, or resolving power, which is the ability to distinguish between two objects. Modern compound light microscopes can only distinguish between objects as close together as 0.2 mm, a distance that is greater than the total diameter of the HSV particle.

It was not until 1931 that major advances led to increased magnification and resolution. Ernst Ruska, a student from the Technical University in Berlin, Germany, hypothesized that electrons focused on a specimen could act like light waves with very short wavelengths, providing the means for greater resolution. Although it took many years to create a working **electron microscope**, Ruska was ultimately successful. Today, electron microscopes magnify objects from 10,000X up to millions of times with excellent resolution, providing views of even the smallest viruses and bacteria (Figure 3.4).

The use of the electron beam prohibits electron microscopic examination of living specimens; this means that samples must be fixed with chemicals and plastic resins in order to be observed with the electron microscope. Cryoelectron microscopy is an alternate form of sample preparation that makes use of a rapid freezing process that stops metabolic processes and preserves biologic structure.

Electron microscopy has been a key development in furthering the science of virology. With virus particles now visible, scientists have been able to understand more about the structure of viruses and their interaction with host cells. For his pioneering development of the electron microscope and the many important scientific discoveries that resulted from it, Ernst Ruska received the Nobel Prize in physics in 1986.

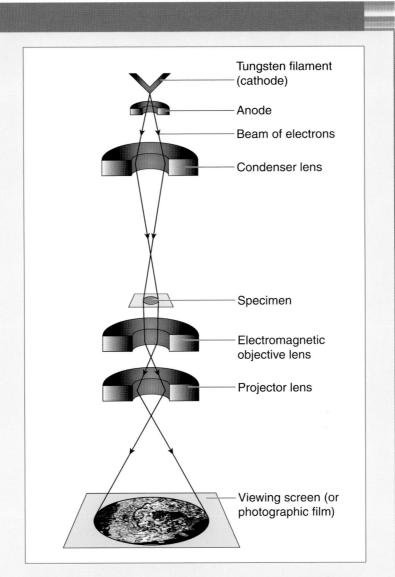

Tungsten filament
(cathode)

Anode

Beam of electrons

Condenser lens

Specimen

Electromagnetic
objective lens

Projector lens

Viewing screen (or
photographic film)

Figure 3.4 This diagram shows the path of an electron beam in a transmission electron microscope. Specimens must be sliced into very thin sections, placed on a copper grid, and stained with heavy metals in order to withstand the bombardment of electrons and allow for a highly magnified image.

(continued from page 35)

proteins provide support for assembly of the capsid, but they are not found in the final infectious virus particle. The way this works is similar to the use of metal scaffold frames that provide support during construction of a new building, but are removed once the structure is nearly completed.

The scaffolding proteins assemble the procapsid, a more fragile precursor capsid that matures into the stable icosahedral shell. Once procapsid assembly is complete, the scaffold is released from the capsid by the action of a viral protease. The protease is an enzyme that severs the attachment between the major capsid protein and the scaffolding proteins, resulting in a mature icosahedral shell that is ready to be packaged with a viral genome. The process of capsid assembly occurs in the nucleus of an infected cell, and once the capsid is packaged with a newly replicated virus genome, it exits the nucleus, acquiring a tegument and envelope on the way out of the cell. A capsid particle that contains a viral genome is called a **nucleocapsid**.

THE TEGUMENT

The tegument is the name used to describe the dense protein structure between the capsid and the envelope. The tegument remains a source of mystery to virologists, who have yet to observe any distinctive features, even with electron microscopic examination. All herpes viruses have a tegument, and the components of this protein layer are known to be involved in regulating activities in the host cell and activating transcription of viral genes. It is believed that tegument proteins perform important functions that aid in establishing virus infection and that their presence in the virus enables them to act in the cell even before the first viral genes are expressed. One of the best-studied tegument proteins is UL48, also known as α-TIF (α-trans-inducing factor), which stimulates expression of immediate early virus genes. The function of many tegument proteins remains unknown.

A VIRUS CAPSID AS A HOME

R. Buckminster Fuller was a scientist and philosopher who gained renown as the inventor and designer of the architectural dome. Fuller wished to apply his technological know-how to one of the most basic and persistent problems of humankind— the lack of efficient, affordable human shelter. Building upon the basic principles of science, his structures made use of tension instead of the usual compression. By way of example, Fuller demonstrated how the difference in strength between a rectangle and a triangle could be confirmed by applying pressure to both structures. While the rectangle would fold up and become unstable, the triangle could withstand the pressure. Fuller's design, the patented geodesic dome (Figure 3.5), was a spherical structure composed of triangles with unparalleled strength. The sphere encloses the largest volume of interior space with the least amount of surface area, which Fuller described as "doing more with less." From a home construction standpoint, this represents a considerable savings on materials and cost.

Fuller further demonstrated that when the sphere's diameter was doubled, it would quadruple the square footage and produce eight times the volume! In addition, the spherical structure of a dome is one of the most efficient designs for a human dwelling because air and energy are allowed to circulate without obstruction. The dome design minimizes exposure to heat in the summer and cold in the winter because of the decreased surface area, which enables heating and cooling to occur naturally.

At the Milan Triennale in 1954, an international exhibition of the most innovative accomplishments in the fields of design, architecture, and city planning, Fuller's dome gained world-wide attention and was awarded the highest honor, the Gran Premio. Since Fuller introduced them, thousands of geodesic shelters have been built all round the world in different climates and temperatures. Although Fuller passed away in 1986, he was honored by the U.S. Postal Service with a commemorative stamp on July 12, 2004, which would have been his 109th birthday.

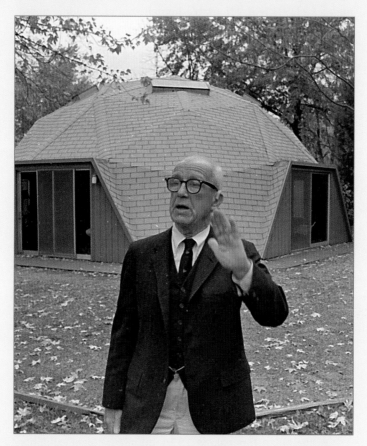

Figure 3.5 Buckminster Fuller stands outside one of his dome homes in 1971. Geodesic dome homes were designed by Fuller to increase interior space and improve heating and cooling efficiency, while decreasing construction costs. Like the virus particles that employ the same design, these geodesic homes were meant to be stable, sturdy, and easily assembled.

THE ENVELOPE

The envelope surrounding the HSV particle is a phospholipid bilayer derived from the host membrane. All biological membranes are composed of two layers of fat molecules called phospholipids because they have two fatty acid chains linked to a phosphate group. Many viruses exit the cell by pushing out through the cell membrane in a process called budding. Because the fatty cell membrane is flexible, it will stretch to a point, then break, and the two segments will reseal, one around the host cell and one around the virus. The virus envelope contains a number of glycoprotein spikes. These glycoproteins are transmembrane proteins, meaning that a portion of the protein projects outside of the membrane, and a portion runs right through it. The part of the protein outside of the membrane is decorated with carbohydrate chains, or sugar residues, in a process known as glycosylation. Membrane proteins with carbohydrates attached are referred to as glycoproteins. The envelope glycoproteins are responsible for the initial contact of HSV with a cell, and they mediate attachment of the virus particle to the surface of the host cell. HSV encodes more than 10 different glycoproteins, but only a subset of these—glycoproteins gB, gD, gH, and gL— is required for virus attachment and entry of the virus particle into the cell. The other viral glycoproteins may aid in the attachment process or facilitate attachment to specific cell types such as neurons, the site of HSV latency.

4

Virus Replication

Imagine Blackbeard the pirate guiding his ship quietly through the night and stealthily up alongside a larger trading vessel. Blackbeard's crew quickly boards the captured ship, taking over the boat and all of the valuable cargo it holds. The process by which a virus infects a cell is actually quite similar to the capture of a ship by pirates. Viruses lack specific treasures (such as metabolic enzymes and equipment for protein synthesis) that can be found in the cell. For a virus to replicate and produce more viruses, it must invade a host cell and take over that host's metabolic machinery. A single virion, or mature virus particle, that infects one cell can give rise to tens, hundreds, or even thousands of new viruses, a process that often leads to the destruction of the cell.

Virus replication involves the following six stages (Figure 4.1):

1. Attachment and entry into the host cell

2. Uncoating of the viral genome

3. Expression of viral genes

4. Replication of the viral genome

5. Assembly of new infectious virions

6. Departure from the infected cell.

Although the same basic steps occur for almost all animal viruses, there is considerable variation in the details. Because herpes viruses are the subject of extensive scientific research, many of the details of HSV

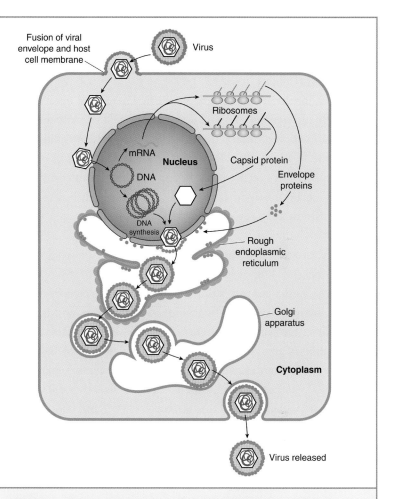

Figure 4.1 Virus replication for HSV is illustrated here. The virus attaches to the potential host cell by binding cell surface receptors, triggering fusion of the viral envelope with the cell membrane. Next, the nucleocapsid travels through the cytoplasm and docks at the nuclear pores, where it releases viral DNA into the nucleus. Transcription of viral genes begins. Viral mRNAs are exported from the nucleus and translated into proteins on host ribosomes. The viral genome is replicated and unit length genomes are packaged into preformed icosahedral capsid shells. The newly formed nucleocapsids exit the nucleus, acquire tegument and envelope proteins, and then exit the cell.

replication have been described at the molecular level. In this chapter, each stage of virus replication is discussed.

ATTACHMENT AND ENTRY

Virus infection begins with a specific interaction between the virus and host cell. Like a key fitting into a lock, only the right combination of interactions will allow the virus to gain access to the host cell. For HSV, glycoproteins on the virus surface interact with specific receptors and **proteoglycans** on the cell surface. Proteoglycans protect tissues in the body by providing a cushion that resists compressive forces. Heparan sulfate proteoglycans are the preferred binding site for infectious HSV particles. The initial contact of HSV with a cell occurs through binding of viral glycoprotein B (gB) or glycoprotein C (gC) to heparan sulfate proteoglycans. However, this interaction is only the first point of attachment, and it is not sufficient to permit virus entry. The next step requires specific binding of the viral glycoprotein D (gD) to one of the entry receptors. There are several possible entry receptors, including HVEM (herpesvirus entry mediator) and two other cell surface proteins called nectin-1 and nectin-2. HSV-1 and HSV-2 differ slightly in their preference for entry receptors. Whereas both HVEM and nectin-1 permit entry by both types of herpes viruses, nectin-2 is exclusive for HSV-2 and is virtually inactive for HSV-1 entry.

Although heparan sulfate proteoglycans are found on almost every cell type in the body, HSV infects mainly skin cells and neurons. The use of multiple receptors for virus entry may allow the virus to enter different cell types; for example, nectin-1 may allow entry into neurons, while HVEM mediates entry into epithelial cells.

Attachment of the virion to the cell surface results in activation of the penetration process. Although the specific events are poorly understood, viral glycoproteins are believed to initiate a fusion between the viral envelope and the cell

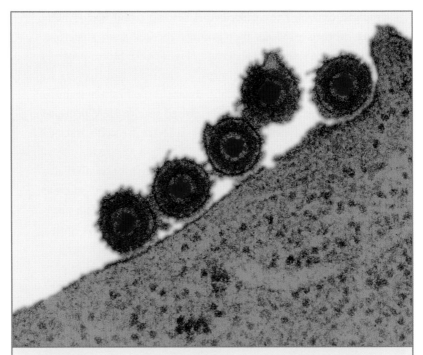

Figure 4.2 Virus particles attached to the surface of a potential host cell can be seen in this electron micrograph. One virus (the one at top right) has engaged the cell surface receptors and begins to enter through the cell membrane.

membrane. When the two membranes fuse into one, the virus nucleocapsid and tegument are released into the host cell's cytoplasm (Figure 4.2).

UNCOATING OF THE VIRAL GENOME

Upon entry into the host cell, some tegument proteins are released into the cytoplasm and some remain associated with the nucleocapsid. The nucleocapsid is transported through the cytoplasm to the nuclear pores, where the viral DNA and selected tegument proteins gain entry to the nucleus. The cellular cytoskeleton mediates transport of the nucleocapsid through the action of the microtubule-associated motor protein, dynein. The cellular cytoskeleton is composed of many long, fibrous proteins that provide the cell with structure, support, and spatial organization (Figure 4.3). Motor proteins like dynein use cellular energy to transport molecules or organelles within the cell along microtubule highways, much like a cargo train traveling on railroad tracks. HSV proteins interact with dynein and hitch a ride to the cell's nucleus along microtubule highways.

The nucleus is enclosed by a double membrane that acts as a barrier between the nucleus and cytoplasm, with **nuclear pores** acting as gateways across that barrier. The nuclear pores are hotbeds of activity, with large numbers of mRNAs exiting and proteins entering the nucleus on a regular basis. The precise mechanism by which the capsid interacts with the nuclear pore is not known, but ultimately the viral DNA is released into the nucleus. Empty capsids have been observed at the nuclear pores early in the infection process. The viral genome is accompanied into the nucleus by a tegument protein, α-trans-inducing factor (α-TIF), which promotes expression of viral genes. Other tegument proteins remain in the cytoplasm to inhibit host protein synthesis.

EXPRESSION OF VIRAL GENES

Transcription of viral DNA occurs in the nucleus of the infected cell, with subsequent protein synthesis occurring in the cytoplasm. The expression of viral genes occurs in a coordinately regulated fashion, with particular functional groups ordered sequentially. The first genes to be expressed are the α-genes, or immediate early genes. Peak synthesis of the protein products of α-genes can be detected within 2 to 4 hours after infection, but the proteins may continue to accumulate during infection at various rates. Of the 75 genes encoded by HSV, only 5 are expressed as α-genes, and they are all believed to have regulatory functions. Functional α-proteins are necessary for the synthesis of β- and γ-gene products.

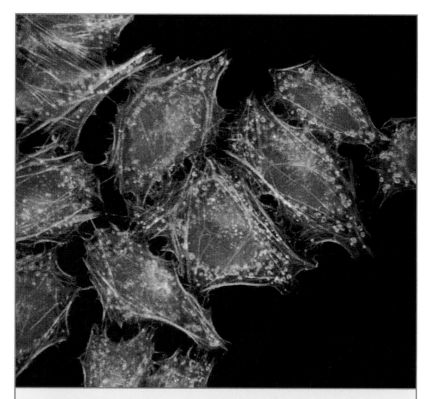

Figure 4.3 This image, taken through an electron microscope, shows the microtubules of the cell cytoskeleton highlighted in green. The microtubule network serves as a railway system for the movement of materials within the cell.

Activation of host cell transcriptional machinery by the α-gene products results in the expression of β-genes, or early genes. The β-gene products include proteins involved in DNA replication and those that aid in nucleic acid metabolism. The appearance of β-gene products coincides with the start of viral DNA replication.

The late genes, or γ-genes, are primarily structural genes. These include capsid proteins, glycoproteins, and tegument proteins, many of which will be packaged into new infectious virions that are released from the cell.

(continued on page 50)

DNA REPLICATION

Replication of DNA is an important process central to all forms of life. When scientists James Watson and Francis Crick described the structure of DNA in 1953, they immediately recognized a potential means for replication of the molecule. Each DNA molecule consists of two long chains coiled together to form a double helix. Each chain has a backbone of sugar molecules connected by phosphate groups, with bases jutting into the center, like rungs on a ladder. Relatively weak bonds hold together two adjacent bases from each chain, so that the entire molecule is effectively "zippered" together into a long double-helical strand. By "unzipping" the molecule, each strand is available to act as a template for synthesis of a new strand. Since there are only four bases present in DNA—adenine, guanine, cytosine, and thymine—there were a limited number of possible combinations. In fact, Watson and Crick determined that adenine always interacted with thymine, and that guanine always interacted with cytosine. As a result, if you knew the sequence of one strand, you could always determine the sequence of what is called the complementary strand.

When replication occurs, the two strands separate (Figure 4.4). The point at which they come apart is generally known as the origin of replication, since it is the site where new DNA synthesis will begin. Synthesis occurs at a replication fork, the point where the two strands are unwound and individual strands are replicated by the addition of complementary bases. The correct bases are added in by an enzyme called DNA poly-merase, which is aided by other proteins that help to unwind the helix and stabilize the resulting single-strands until they are replicated. Generally, the two replication forks move outward from the origin until the entire molecule is copied; however, some bacteria and viruses use an alternative method called **rolling circle replication** (see Figure 4.5 on page 51). Rolling circle replication is especially useful for viruses, because it allows for the rapid, continuous production of many genomes.

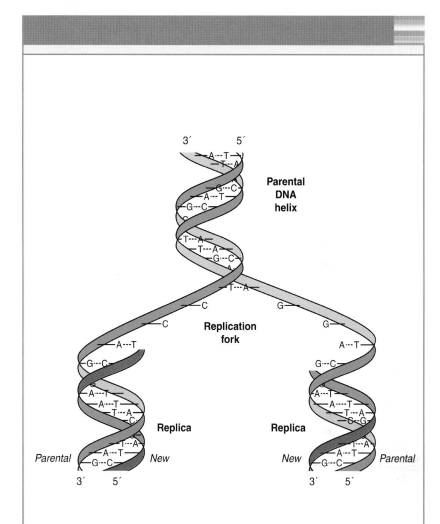

Figure 4.4 DNA replication occurs when the two strands of the double helix unwind. Each strand serves as a template for the addition of complementary bases, which is accomplished through the action of a DNA polymerase and accessory proteins. Ultimately, two strands are produced that are each exact copies of the original strand.

(continued from page 47)

REPLICATION OF THE VIRAL GENOME

Upon entry into the nucleus, the linear viral DNA genome takes on a circular shape through interactions at the ends of the molecule, where the terminal repeat sequences are found. Once the genome has circularized, DNA replication proceeds through the rolling circle method. Commonly used by bacteriophages (viruses that infect bacteria), rolling circle replication allows many genomes to be produced rapidly (Figure 4.5). Viral DNA replication can proceed so rapidly that the origins of the newly replicated strands may also serve as sites of initiation for DNA replication, so that a highly complex linked network of DNA is formed in the nucleus of the infected cell.

DNA replication is a critical event in virus infection. Once a cell begins high-level DNA replication, it is committed to producing new infectious virus particles, a circumstance that generally leads to the host cell's death.

ASSEMBLY OF NEW INFECTIOUS VIRIONS

More than 30 HSV gene products are structural components of the virion. Capsid proteins synthesized in the cytoplasm must enter the nucleus for the process of capsid assembly. The major capsid protein binds to the scaffolding protein, which escorts the major capsid protein through the nuclear pores and into the nucleus. As described in Chapter 3, the major capsid protein assembles on the scaffold. A single infected cell can produce so many capsids that they form what looks like a crystalline array inside the nucleus (Figure 4.6). As the rate of capsid production reaches its highest levels, many of the capsids never even mature and become packaged with DNA; instead, they simply remain in the nucleus with the scaffold still intact.

DEPARTURE FROM THE INFECTED CELL

As the capsid leaves the nucleus, it must acquire tegument proteins, an envelope, and glycoprotein spikes in order to become an infectious virus particle. Some tegument proteins,

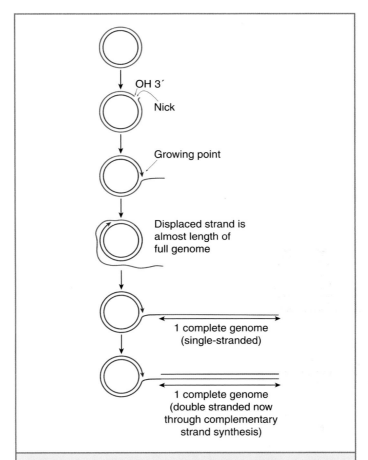

Figure 4.5 Rolling circle replication is a method for rapidly duplicating the circular DNA genomes of some types of bacteria and viruses. Replication begins when one strand is nicked and separated from the other strand. New nucleotide bases are added to the end of the nicked strand (seen at top of this diagram), creating a replacement for the original strand, which is further displaced. As replication continues, a single-stranded copy of the complete length of the genome trails off the end of the circle. The complementary sequence is added, generating a double-stranded complete genome that will eventually be cleaved and will form a circle, forming an exact copy of the original circular genome. Many copies can be made rapidly using this method.

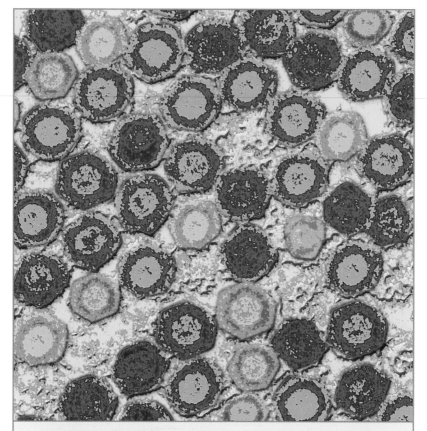

Figure 4.6 Hundreds of virus capsids can accumulate in the nucleus of an infected cell. At times, the density of capsids can become so high that the capsids look much like a tightly packed collection of crystals inside the cell, as seen here.

like α-TIF, bind to the capsid while it is still in the nucleus. Other tegument proteins may be added at other sites, such as the cytoplasm or the endoplasmic reticulum. The **endoplasmic reticulum** is a membranous network that is connected to the nuclear envelope and is a major site of synthesis for proteins that are destined to be secreted or embedded in a membrane. Viral glycoproteins are produced using the cellular machinery in the endoplasmic reticulum, where they are decorated with

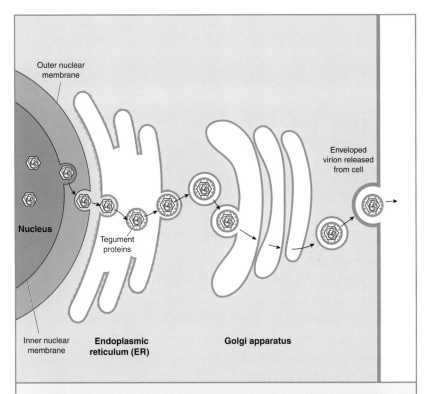

Figure 4.7 HSV capsids are assembled and packaged with viral DNA in the nucleus of infected cells. Newly formed nucleocapsids bud through the nuclear membrane into the cell cytoplasm. The capsid enters the endoplasmic reticulum (ER), where tegument proteins are added. The tegument-coated capsid exits the ER, acquiring glycoproteins from the ER membrane and Golgi apparatus. The enveloped capsid is released from the cell as an infectious particle.

the appropriate sugar molecules. Glycoproteins sent to the plasma membrane become incorporated into the virion as capsids are budding out of the cell. Other glycoproteins remain in the endoplasmic reticulum and associate with the capsid in transport vesicles that are pinched off and ultimately merge with the plasma membrane as the capsid exits the cell (Figure 4.7).

5

Lying in Wait: Virus Latency

The following letter appeared in a local newspaper:

Dear Heloise,

Help, I can't get rid of roaches! I've tried so many chemicals the family and pets should be dead. I can't afford a monthly fee to have someone come in all the time. I've emptied every cupboard and have sprayed, powdered and sealed. Nothing works. They leave during the day but at night are back and it seems they bring more friends. My walls, baseboards and cupboards are being ruined by the constant spraying. Is there any help out there? Thanks!

Disgusted Donna

The reason many people have problems getting rid of roaches is that the roaches usually have a nest somewhere hidden away from the spots where you see them. The nest is a constant source of new roaches waiting to invade your home, since this is the location to which they keep going back to breed, sleep, and maintain their insect colony.

Like a nest of roaches, HSV also establishes a site where viruses are maintained until the time is right for another infection. This phenomenon is known as latency, a period in which viral DNA is present, but no infectious virus particles are being produced.

Latency is one of the defining properties of all herpes viruses. The ability of these viruses to remain latent in the host for its lifetime is one of the most unique and challenging aspects of herpes virus biology. HSV is a **neurotropic** virus, meaning that it can establish latent infection in

(continued on page 57)

The nervous system regulates all aspects of bodily function. It consists of billions of neurons, cells that are designed for the transmission of information between the brain and the rest of the body (Figure 5.1). The structure of a neuron is highly specialized. The cell body contains the nucleus and the majority of ribosomes that serve as sites of protein synthesis. Projecting from the cell body is a single axon, which conducts an electrical impulse, called an action potential, from the cell body to the axon's end, or terminus. The axon terminus is generally close to one or more neurons that receive the signal and transmit it further. Signals are received by dendrites, multiple extensions from the cell body that convert the chemical signal from the axon terminus of one neuron to an electrical impulse that can be sent down the axon.

Sensory neurons receive signals from the environment, such as light, touch, sound, and smell, and pass this information to the brain for processing and storage. Motor neurons regulate the contraction of muscles and the secretion of hormones. The highly specialized nature of nerve cells is due to the expression of genes associated with the nerve cell lineage, a process known as differentiation. As a cell becomes more highly specialized, it no longer undergoes cell division. Because of their important role in regulating bodily functions, nerve cells in particular are stable and long-lived. These properties also make nerve cells an excellent hiding place for a virus. Nerve cells are located throughout the body, giving viruses easy access from almost any site of primary infection. Neurons are so essential to our being that they are rarely attacked by the immune system, and since they do not often divide, there is no need for viral genomes to be replicated and sorted into daughter cells. The treatment of neurological disorders has been hampered by the difficulties of accessing nerve cells and delivering therapeutics (remedies or medications) to them, making it unlikely that there will ever be a way to eradicate latent HSV from neurons. Human beings are a highly evolved species, but HSV has been evolving right along with us and has chosen an exquisite method for making sure it continues to do so.

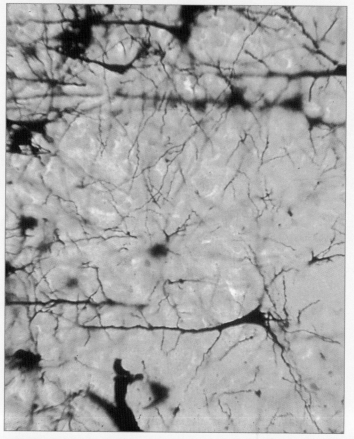

Figure 5.1 Shown here is a network of nerve cells from the brain magnified 100 times.

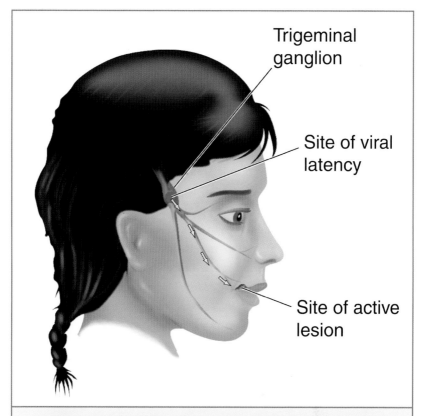

Trigeminal
ganglion

Site of viral
latency

Site of active
lesion

Figure 5.2 The trigeminal ganglion is a bundle of nerves located on the side of the face near the temple. Viruses can leave the epithelial cells and enter the individual neurons that connect to the area. Once inside a neuron, HSV particles can establish lifelong latent infection.

(continued from page 54)

neurons, or nerve cells. Following productive infection of epithelial cells (the cells that cover the body's surface and line bodily cavities), the virus enters sensory neurons that inner-vate the cells of the mucous membranes. A bundle of nerve cells located outside the spinal cord is called a ganglion; HSV-1 establishes latency in the trigeminal ganglion near the face (Figure 5.2), while HSV-2 latency is most commonly estab-lished in the sacral ganglion near the genital region.

A neuron (Figure 5.3) has a cell body, which contains the nucleus, and fiber-like processes of two types: axons and dendrites. Dendrites receive signals from other neurons, while axons convey messages from the neuron to other cells. HSV enters the neuron through the end of the axon near the site of initial infection. Upon entry into the nerve cell, the nucleo-capsid and some associated tegument proteins are rapidly transported to the cell body by the process of **retrograde axonal transport**. Retrograde transport is the movement of cellular materials from the axon to the cell body. It is called "retrograde" because it is the opposite of **anterograde transport**, or the movement of materials in the neuron from the cell body toward the axon. This retrograde transport is a crucial step in the virus life cycle, because without transportation to the cell nucleus, no latency or neuronal replication can occur. Scientists have observed HSV capsids moving in a retrograde direction after injection into a giant squid axon, and the movement has been clocked at 3 to 5 mm per hour.

After traveling up the axon to the cell body, the virus capsid arrives at the nucleus of neuron, where the viral DNA is released through the nuclear pores. The linear DNA genome circularizes and is then maintained as an extra-chromosomal piece of circular DNA called an **episome**. A given neuron may contain 20 to 100 episomal copies of the HSV genome. Although scientists first speculated that this was due to more than one viral genome entering a single neuron during the establish-ment of latency, the current thinking is that viral genomes are replicated by the host cell. Since the nerve cell is fully differentiated and no longer undergoing cell divisions, the viral DNA can persist in the neuron's nucleus for the life of the host.

There are many aspects of HSV latency that remain unclear, and many questions still to be answered. For example, how does the viral genome decide when to reactivate? And when it does reactivate, what initiates the transcription of viral genes? What is known is that reactivation from a latently

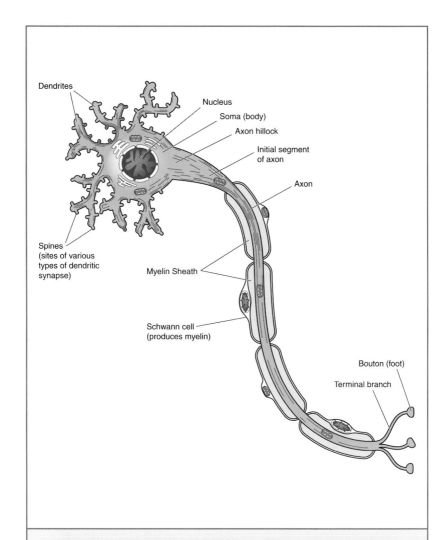

Figure 5.3 This diagram illustrates a nerve cell, depicting the cell body, where the nucleus is located, and the dendrites and axon. The dendrites receive signals from other neurons, while the long axon sends signals to adjacent neurons or muscle cells. The axon is insulated by Schwann cells that form a myelin sheath, which helps nerve impulses move more quickly. HSV particles enter a neuron at the axon terminus and travel by retrograde transport to the cell body, where the viral genome is maintained in the nucleus.

infected neuron involves a highly orchestrated series of interactions between viral genes. It is believed that limited replication occurs in the nucleus of the neuron, resulting in the production of nucleocapsid particles. These nucleocapsids

THE HUMAN IMMUNE SYSTEM: WHY CAN'T IT STOP HSV?

Like a well-trained army, the immune system monitors our body for the presence of foreign invaders. It does an excellent job of stopping rogue pollen grains, bacteria, and viruses from causing us serious harm, most of the time. Why, then, is the immune system so ineffective at stopping HSV, a microscopic particle that acts more like a massive tank than the tiny piece of DNA and protein that it is?

Chinese philosopher Sun Tzu's *The Art of War* describes how to think about challenges in a new way, not as fighting others, but as advancing your own position to make success inevitable. HSV has mastered this through the art of immune evasion. The secret to the success of this tiny guerrilla warrior is that it is has numerous strategies for thwarting offensive maneuvers by the immune system. For example, a virus-infected cell is usually identified by circulating lymphocytes, cells that defend the body against dangerous invaders, because of a tag displayed on the cell surface. The tag is composed of cellular proteins, called major histocompatibility complexes (MHC), that bind to small bits of virus capsid proteins that have entered the cell. Since the capsid proteins are foreign, the cell is identified as infected and lymphocytes known as killer T cells destroy it. Since recognition depends on MHC proteins being displayed on the cell surface, HSV destabilizes MHC proteins and prevents them from being expressed on the cell surface, effectively subverting immune surveillance.

are then transported back down from the cell body to the axon via anterograde transport, where they can infect mucosal epithelial cells again.

Although the molecular mechanisms governing HSV latency remain unknown, it is clear that reactivation can happen many times, with no apparent damage to the ganglia. It is not known whether one or even several neurons die with each reactivation, but there are so many neurons in the ganglia that there have been no reported cases of lost sensation in the lips or sacral region among people with recurrent infection. In some unknown way, HSV can determine when the conditions

APOPTOSIS: PROGRAMMED CELL DEATH

"Ask not what your country can do for you; ask what you can do for your country," President John F. Kennedy said in his inspiring inaugural address to the nation in 1961. In the body, one of every ten individuals is asked to make a sacrifice for the greater good. In a multicellular organism, cells are occasionally called upon to make the ultimate sacrifice. Cell suicide is an odd sort of fate, but one that is nonetheless essential to our overall development. Cell suicide is scientifically termed *apoptosis*, or programmed cell death, and it keeps our hands from being webbed and our immune system from attacking our own tissues and proteins.

Apoptosis comes from a Greek word that means "dropping off" or "falling off," as leaves do from a tree. Dying cells shrink and condense through a series of specific and ordered cellular events. This is quite different from cells that die by **necrosis**, a response to tissue damage in which cells swell and burst, releasing their contents and potentially damaging surrounding cells. In contrast, fragments of the dying apoptotic cell are usually engulfed by other cells, and in the end, there is virtually no evidence that the cell ever existed at all (Figure 5.4).

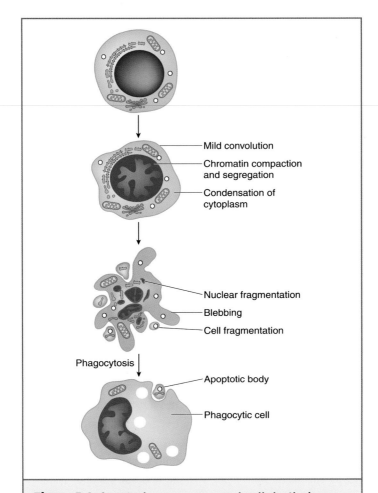

Figure 5.4 Apoptosis, or programmed cell death, is an ordered series of events that leads to the complete removal of the selected cell. In response to death signals, a cell-signaling cascade is activated, resulting in condensation of the cell and fragmentation of the cellular DNA. Ultimately, the cell fragments are engulfed by phagocytic white blood cells and all traces of the cell are gone.

in the host are right, and the latent virus can shift to productive infection in which the infectious virus may be transmitted to other susceptible individuals.

6

Clinical Syndromes

If you've ever watched television shows like *ER* or *Chicago Hope*, you know that patients can unexpectedly develop serious complications. Although the skin lesions caused by HSV can range from mild or even unnoticeable to large patches of painful blisters, they are usually not life-threatening and generally go away within a few days, leaving little evidence of the outbreak. However, in some cases of HSV infection, more severe, life-threatening disease can result. In this chapter, the various clinical manifestations of herpes virus infection are discussed.

ORAL INFECTION

The most frequent clinical manifestations of primary infection with HSV-1 are gingivostomatitis and pharyngitis. The infections can range from totally asymptomatic to combinations of fever, sore throat, swollen glands, and vesicular lesions. **Gingivostomatitis** is a condition in which sores are present on the mouth and gums (Figure 6.1), which can cause difficulty eating. If the lesions are present on the lips, they have a tendency to crust over, whereas lesions inside the mouth or on the gums do not. In individuals who are exposed to HSV during adolescence rather than during early childhood, HSV **pharyngitis**, or inflammation of the pharynx (throat), is becoming a more common diagnosis, sometimes in conjunction with mononucleosis. The incubation period for oral herpes infections, the amount of time between contact with the virus and the appearance of symptoms, ranges from 2 to 12 days, meaning that the lesions contain infectious virus for this time period. People who experience recurrent outbreaks can usually tell when they are about to occur due to the presence of tingling, burning, or itching at the site of the upcoming outbreak. These

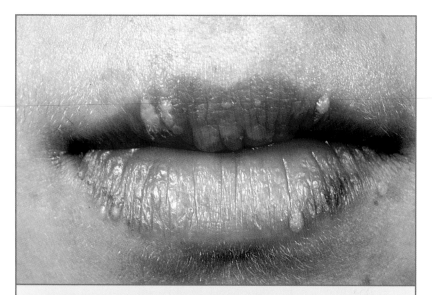

Figure 6.1 HSV infection of epithelial cells in the face and mouth can lead to the formation of small, painful blisters, as seen on this person's lips.

are termed **prodromal** symptoms. Pain is most severe at the outset of the outbreak and resolves quickly within a few days. Healing is generally rapid, and there is little or no specific treatment for oral herpes outbreaks.

EYE INFECTION

HSV infection of the eye may be initiated by the transfer of virus from a cold sore to the eye. **Herpetic keratitis** is a sight-threatening condition that may manifest after some sort of trauma to the eye, such as a scratch or sunburn. The infection causes irritation and excessive tearing, but is relatively pain-less. Generally, only one eye is affected, and in many cases, the infection will go away without causing permanent damage. However, in some cases, the infection is more severe, and lesions, or tears, can occur in the cornea so that deeper tissue layers may be infected, resulting in corneal scarring and

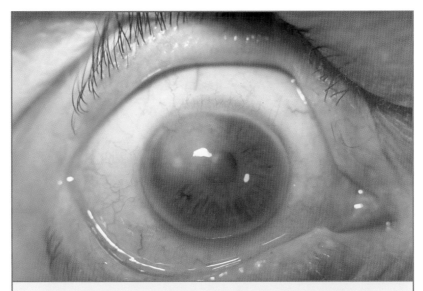

Figure 6.2 Infection of the eye with HSV can lead to ulceration of the cornea and could lead to blindness unless properly treated.

ultimately vision impairment (Figure 6.2). Even more severe damage can occur in the event of a misdiagnosis that results in prescription of eyedrops containing steroids. The steroids suppress immune function and can exacerbate the infection, leading to corneal destruction and blindness. The presence of typical herpes blisters on the eyelids may aid in diagnosis, but they do not always occur. The infection may be treated with eyedrops containing antiviral agents, but the patient is likely to suffer recurrent bouts, and herpetic keratitis is currently a leading cause of blindness in the United States. Vision may be restored only with a corneal transplant, and a large percentage of the corneal transplants currently performed are to treat corneal scarring from HSV.

SKIN INFECTION

HSV can establish infections of the skin through small cuts or abrasions on the skin surface. **Herpetic whitlow** (Figure 6.3)

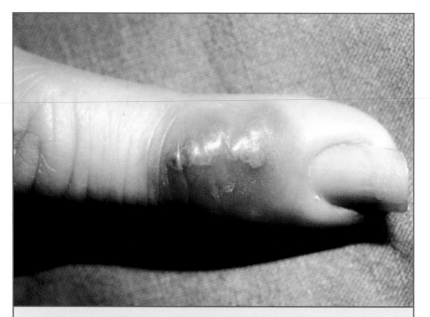

Figure 6.3 Herpetic whitlow (seen here) can occur on the fingers or hands. It usually results when virus from the face or genitals enters through small breaks in the skin.

is an intense painful infection of the hand involving one or more fingers. It is relatively common in young children with cold sores who suck their thumbs or bite their fingers. Doctors and nurses who provide care for HSV-infected patients are also at risk for accidental infection. In these cases of herpetic whitlow, the agent is generally HSV-1. In adolescents with genital herpes, however, herpetic whitlow can be caused by HSV-2. This is due to itching and scratching of the genital lesions, which can result in infection on the hands through small cuts or breaks in the skin. Pain and swelling occur, and pustular vesicles develop. Primary lesions may take up to three weeks to heal. Recurrent episodes are common, and these tend to heal more quickly.

Another form of HSV skin infection is **herpes gladiatorum**, a condition that is common in athletes engaged in contact sports, such as wrestlers and rugby players. In this condition, lesions are present on other skin surfaces, especially the chest.

A severe form of herpes that affects the skin can also occur in children with active eczema. In patients with **eczema herpeticum**, chicken pox–like vesicles may appear in the areas already affected by eczema. The resulting disease can be quite serious, resulting in protein loss and dehydration. Because the underlying eczema promotes the spread of the infection along the skin and to other sites such as the liver or adrenal glands, the condition can be fatal. Patients with severe burns may also be at risk of eczema herpeticum. Early diagnosis and rapid antiviral therapy are the keys to managing the infection.

CENTRAL NERVOUS SYSTEM INFECTIONS

Given the propensity of HSV for latent infection in neurons, it is not unexpected that infections of the brain occur. Fortunately, while extremely serious and potentially deadly, these forms of infection are rare. *Encephalitis* is defined as inflammation of brain tissue. **Herpes encephalitis** is the most common form of sporadic viral encephalitis in the United States. It is an acute illness with a high mortality rate. The onset of the disease may include a period of fever and malaise, followed by neurological symptoms such as headaches and behavioral changes. This stage is often followed by a seizure or sudden paralysis, which can give way to coma and ultimately death. Early recognition and specific antiviral therapy are the keys to survival, but the treatment must be started as soon as possible and before the patient progresses to the coma stage. The risk factors that lead to herpes encephalitis remain unknown. It can occur at any time of year and in patients of any age, although the condition is slightly more frequent among people who are 50 to 70 years old. Usually, there is some evidence of previous HSV infection, but recurrent lesions are almost never seen at the time of disease onset. HSV-1 is most often the causative agent, but HSV-2 does occur in those with compromised immune systems, especially HIV-positive individuals or persons with AIDS.

Another complication of genital herpes infection is **HSV meningitis**. Meningitis is an inflammation of the meninges, the membranes protecting the brain and spinal cord. Swelling around the brain produces increased pressure inside the skull, generally resulting in intense headaches. Inflammation of the spinal meninges can affect nearby muscles and cause a stiff neck, another classic symptom of meningitis. Meningitis can be caused by a number of different bacterial, viral, and even fungal pathogens, with bacterial meningitis causing the most serious and life-threatening disease. When a patient with typical symptoms of meningitis is found to have no bacteria present in the cerebrospinal fluid, viral infection is the presumed cause. Viral meningitis accounts for about 40% of all cases of meningitis; fortunately, it is far less serious than bacterial meningitis and usually goes away within a week. Many viruses can cause meningitis. In a patient known to have genital herpes, HSV-2 is the presumed cause.

NEONATAL HERPES

Neonatal herpes is a devastating and frequently fatal disease affecting newborn infants infected with the herpes simplex virus (HSV). Almost always caused by HSV-2, infection of the newborn occurs during passage through the birth canal if the mother is actively shedding virus at the time of the delivery. If the mother has a primary infection, the transmission rate is very high. With recurrent infection, transmission rates are significantly lower. It is difficult to prevent neonatal herpes because the majority of women have no symptoms and no clinical history of genital herpes. Neonatal herpes usually becomes evident about six days after birth. Because the infant lacks a developed immune system, the infection can rapidly spread to the liver, lungs, and even the central nervous system (CNS). Once the CNS is infected, death is imminent, and

GENITAL HERPES AND HIV: DOUBLE TROUBLE

Patients with one type of sexually transmitted disease are very likely to have additional infections. One reason for this is simply that the risk factors are the same and behaviors that lead to infection with one STD, such as having intercourse with multiple partners or without a condom, make it easier to spread other STDs. With genital herpes, there is additional risk for contracting human immunodeficiency virus (HIV). Because genital herpes infection can result in open sores, the skin no longer provides an effective barrier against infection, and HIV has direct access to the bloodstream. People with an active genital herpes infection are much more likely to contract HIV than those without genital lesions. Interestingly, those with a more recent incident of primary genital herpes infection (within the past six months) have twice the risk of becoming infected with HIV. This appears to be mainly because reactivation rates tend to be two to three times higher in the first six months after primary infection.

Once an individual is doubly infected with HSV and HIV, more serious problems can result. Although HSV can cause recurrent painful blisters, the disease is generally relatively benign. In classic cases, the vesicles rupture, crust over, and then heal. Recurrent infections that result from latent stores of the virus in neurons are generally not life-threatening. In HIV-positive individuals, however, the frequency and severity of outbreaks increase, in part due to the immune suppression caused by the destruction of lymphocytes by the HIV virus. Although herpes infections are not included in the definition of AIDS, it is still possible for serious herpes-related complications, such as meningitis or keratitis, to arise in patients with HIV.

the fatality rate for untreated neonatal herpes is greater than 60%. Even with treatment, many survivors suffer permanent mental retardation or neurologic disability. As with other complications due to herpes, early antiviral therapy is the key to survival.

Occasionally, herpes virus transmission to the newborn can also occur after delivery by direct contact with infected family members or hospital personnel. In these cases, the clinical symptoms and outcomes of the disease are the same, but the infection is more likely due to HSV-1.

7

Diagnosis and Treatment

Matt is disturbed to find that he has a cluster of small painful blisters on his penis. They appeared several days after he had a sexual encounter with a young woman he met at a club. He has been surfing the Internet and is pretty sure he has genital herpes. All the information he's found says there is no cure for the disease, so he wonders why he should even bother seeing the doctor. He's not planning to see the woman again, and he doesn't want his parents or friends to find out about his condition. Besides, he thinks, the blisters should go away soon, and they aren't life-threatening, right?

Contrary to Matt's reasoning, it is very important to consult a physician if you suspect you have genital herpes, for several reasons. First, if the infection is severe, it can be very painful, and there are medications available to lessen the severity of the outbreak. Second, if there is a chance you have been exposed to HSV, the possibility also exists that you could have contracted other STDs. While there is no cure available for genital herpes, many other infections, like chlamydia and gonorrhea, can easily be treated with antibiotics. Even worse, if untreated, chlamydia and gonorrhea can lead to serious disease, particularly in women. Pelvic inflammatory disease, an infection of the upper genital tract, is a common result of untreated STD infections and a leading cause of infertility among young women today. Finally, your physician should take a few moments to explain to you that even if you do have genital herpes, you can still lead a normal life and have healthy sexual relationships, provided you take precautions (Figure 7.1).

DIAGNOSIS

Suppose Matt decides to visit an STD clinic for an accurate diagnosis and treatment. The diagnosis of an STD usually begins with a series of questions

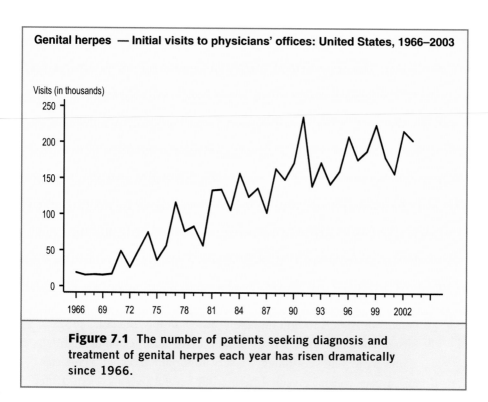

Genital herpes — Initial visits to physicians' offices: United States, 1966–2003

Visits (in thousands)

Figure 7.1 The number of patients seeking diagnosis and treatment of genital herpes each year has risen dramatically since 1966.

for the patient. The doctor or nurse practitioner will probably begin by asking about the specific reason for the visit. In addition to hearing a description of the current symptoms, he or she will also ask whether there have been any similar symptoms before. The patient can expect to be asked questions about his or her sexual behavior and history. The number of sexual partners, a recent change in sexual partners, and whether or not condoms were used are all important information.

Next, the doctor will need to perform a thorough physical examination. For women, this will mean a pelvic exam, so that the cervix and vagina can be inspected. The area between the vulva and the anus should also be carefully examined for signs of infection. For men, the exam will include a close-up look at the penis, scrotum, and rectum. In each case, the doctor will be looking for blisters or skin lesions characteristic of genital

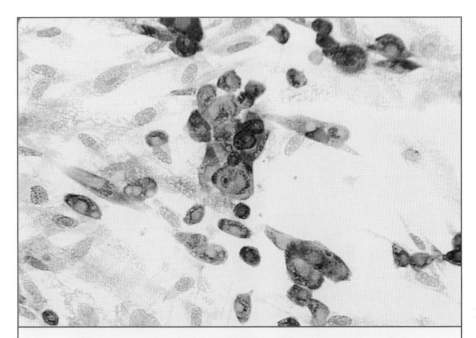

Figure 7.2 Cells infected with HSV exhibit a rounded morphology, generally visible 1 to 5 days after infection with the virus.

herpes. For both men and women, swabs from the genitalia will most likely be taken for a laboratory test (Figure 7.2).

THE LABORATORY TESTS

The gold standard laboratory test for HSV diagnosis is a viral culture. However, the viral culture can take up to 10 days to display signs of infection, and sometimes even very good samples from herpes lesions may be negative (when a culture is positive but tests negative, this is called a "false-negative" test). Vesicles and wet lesions are more likely to contain infectious virus than dry, crusty ones. Unfortunately, many patients don't have lesions when they go to the doctor, and more than half of patient samples from a recurrent episode (rather than the primary infection) test negative. Negative tests often result because the recurrent infection is milder and fewer lesions and fewer infectious virus particles may be present. Another drawback of the culture is that a positive result can clearly indicate HSV, but it will not indicate whether the infection is caused by HSV-1 or HSV-2.

Serology, or blood testing, may be used for patients who don't exhibit lesions. This test determines, based on the presence of antibodies in the bloodstream, if the patient has previously been exposed to the herpes virus. Antibodies are proteins generated by the immune system to recognize and combat foreign invaders, and most people who have been infected will have HSV-specific antibodies. Serological testing is advised even in the event of a positive viral culture test, since this method can distinguish between HSV-1 and HSV-2. Identification of the specific type of HSV is helpful for the physician for accurate epidemiology data and for the patient because HSV-1 tends to cause less frequent and milder recurrent outbreaks than HSV-2.

One drawback of the serology test is that a patient may test negative for the herpes virus if the test is performed very soon after initial exposure. If the patient has a primary herpes infection, it can take weeks or even months to develop antibodies to the virus. Unfortunately, the primary outbreaks usually have the most severe symptoms and this is the most likely time for the patient to consult a physician.

TREATMENT

Although there is no cure for herpes infection, treatment with the drug acyclovir (Figure 7.3) is very effective at shortening or preventing outbreaks. The brand name for acyclovir is Zovirax®, and a physician may prescribe it or a related drug, such as famciclovir (Famvir®) or valacyclovir (Valtrex®) to treat a primary infection. The treatment is most effective when the medication is started within 2 days of the onset of symptoms, but it may still help alleviate symptoms even if started up to a week after the onset of the outbreak. The

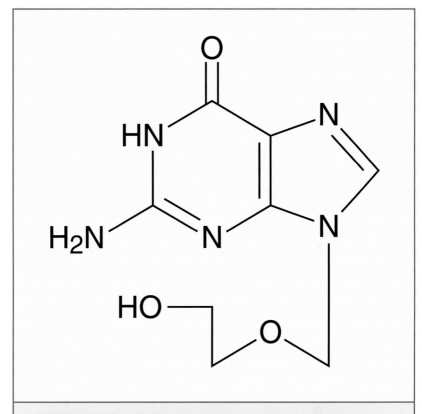

Figure 7.3 This illustration shows the chemical structure of acyclovir, a potent antiviral therapeutic. Inside infected cells, acyclovir is modified by viral enzymes, which causes viral DNA replication to stop.

course of treatment is generally 7 to 10 days. Acyclovir is taken five times a day, while valacyclovir and famciclovir are both taken twice a day.

If the individual is prone to recurrent episodes, the doctor may prescribe acyclovir for treatment during the prodromal period (the period before symptoms occur) or immediately after the onset of symptoms. Episodic treatment generally requires a 5-day course of medication. Patients with very severe or frequent recurrences may be treated with suppressive

(continued on page 78)

PRINCIPLES OF DRUG DISCOVERY

Acyclovir remains one of the most resounding success stories in the history of drug discovery. Acyclovir is a chemical that was specifically designed to inhibit herpes virus replication. The structure of acyclovir is similar to the structure of a nucleotide building block that would be used to replicate DNA in a dividing cell. By altering the structure of normal nucleotides, scientists at Burroughs Wellcome set out to develop chemical compounds that would inhibit the process of DNA synthesis in cancer cells, bacteria, and viruses without affecting the growth of normal cells in the body. Gertrude Elion (Figure 7.4) and George Hitchings were awarded the 1988 Nobel Prize in Physiology or Medicine, along with Sir James Black, for their contributions to the science of drug development for the treatment of a variety of serious illnesses, including leukemia, transplant rejection, and HSV infection.

When a patient takes acyclovir, the molecules enter cells and are selectively modified by a viral enzyme called thymidine kinase. The thymidine kinase converts acyclovir to an active compound, acyclovir triphosphate. The acyclovir triphosphate looks chemically similar to the normal nucleotide triphosphates that are added to growing DNA chains during replication by DNA polymerases. Since HSV uses its own viral DNA polymerase for replication instead of borrowing the cellular enzymes like many other viruses do, the viral DNA polymerase became a prime target for drug development. Acyclovir competes with normal nucleotides for incorporation into the DNA strands that are newly formed during replication. There's just one problem—acyclovir lacks the chemical group, called the 3'-hydroxyl, to which the next nucleotide in the sequence would be added. As a result, acyclovir is also called a chain terminator, because after it is added, no further nucleotides can be attached and DNA synthesis stops. The result is specific inhibition of viral

DNA replication, with little effect on the host cell. Compounds that act as chain terminators have also been developed that successfully inhibit replication of HIV.

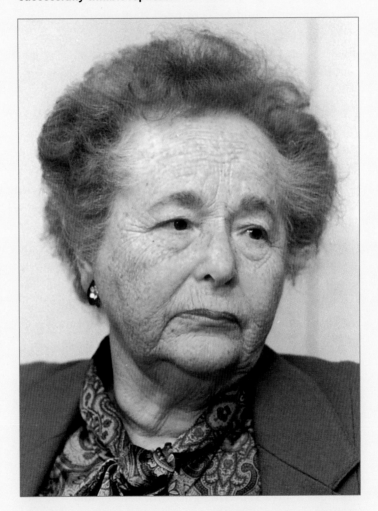

Figure 7.4 Gertrude Elion won the 1988 Nobel Prize in Physiology or Medicine for work that led to the development of therapeutics for leukemia and HSV infection.

(continued from page 75)

therapy. Suppressive therapy involves taking antiviral medication every day for an extended period of time, such as several months or a year. The aim is to reduce the frequency of occurrences and to lessen the severity of the outbreaks. After several months, the doctor will review whether or not the treatment should be continued. Individuals who have more than six outbreaks a year, who have extremely painful episodes, or who are experiencing depression or anxiety due to recurrent outbreaks are candidates for suppressive therapy.

Patients on suppressive therapy should be aware that just because their outbreaks become milder or occur less often does not mean they are no longer infectious. Suppressive therapy does not necessarily reduce the risk of transmitting HSV to a sexual partner. It is still important to use condoms or refrain from sexual intercourse when lesions are present in order to protect a partner from contracting genital herpes.

Acyclovir and related drugs have minimal toxicity, meaning that they are usually well tolerated by patients and no major side effects have been reported. Some patients experience minor side effects, such as headache, nausea, and diarrhea. Acyclovir is safe and effective, and has no known interactions with other drugs. Although it is usually administered orally for treatment of patients with genital herpes, acyclovir may also be given intravenously (by a needle in a vein) for patients with serious conditions such as herpes encephalitis. The drug is effective against HSV-1, HSV-2, and varicella zoster virus.

Topical formulations of acyclovir are also available for direct application to skin lesions, but there is some debate among physicians about whether or not this is really beneficial. In addition, dozens of Websites have appeared on the Internet in the past few years advertising herbal or homeopathic remedies for herpes infection. None of these remedies has been scientifically shown to relieve symptoms; when in doubt, it is best to consult with your physician.

8

Prevention and Control

Imagine laughing and running or playing soccer with your friends one day, and then becoming paralyzed the next. In the early 1950s, this was a very real fear as polio, a serious neurological disease, swept across the United States, crippling thousands of once healthy and active children. In 1952 alone, infection with the poliovirus caused nearly 40,000 cases of paralytic polio and more than 3,000 deaths.

Poliovirus had been around for many years, but improved sanitation changed the way the population was exposed to the virus. Previously, people had often been exposed to open sewers and other unsanitary conditions, and the poliovirus present in fecal waste caused mild or asymptomatic infections in infants or very young children (when paralysis is rare). These children then developed lifelong immunity. As sewage treatment improved, people no longer experienced the mild infection and immunity at a young age. Instead, older children and adults with no prior immunity might be exposed and the disease would grow from a very mild, uncommon occurrence to a terrifying epidemic. Fortunately, the epidemic was brought under control through the efforts of a microbiologist named Jonas Salk (Figure 8.1). Salk developed a chemically inactivated form of the poliovirus that could be used as a **vaccine**, an agent that provides immunity without causing disease. People who were treated with the inactivated poliovirus vaccine didn't get sick, but they did mount an immune response to the virus that would protect them in case they were ever exposed to infectious virus. Later, the Sabin vaccine, which consisted of a live, **attenuated** (weakened) virus, became more widely used, since it resulted in a longer-lasting immune response. Today, polio has been eradicated in the United States, and vaccination will continue until it has been eradicated worldwide.

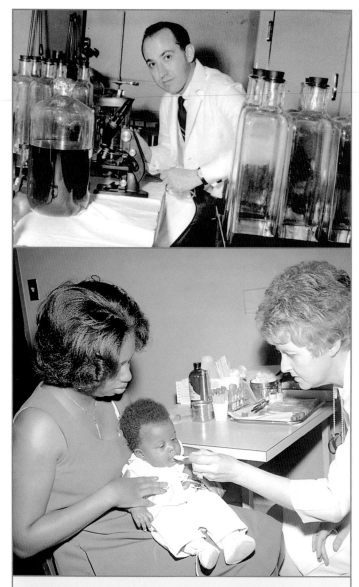

Figure 8.1 Top: Dr. Jonas Salk works with his microscope at Pittsburgh's Municipal Hospital Laboratory after the announcement of his successful polio vaccine on April 18, 1955. Bottom: An infant receives the polio vaccine via oral administration.

The development of the poliovirus vaccine was a huge success, and since the 1950s, successful vaccines for several diseases have been produced. Despite the many advances in medical research and human health care, it has proven difficult to develop safe and effective vaccines for many other serious diseases. With more than 45 million people affected in the United States alone, genital herpes remains one of the diseases for which no vaccine exists.

Research is under way, however, and a collaborative effort between the National Institutes of Allergy and Infectious Disease (a part of the National Institutes of Health) and pharmaceutical company GlaxoSmithKline could make the first HSV vaccine available soon. The Herpevac Trial for Women is a research study investigating a vaccine that may protect women against genital herpes. With 23 study sites around the country, more than 7,000 women will randomly be assigned to receive either the candidate herpes vaccine or another investigational vaccine directed against the hepatitis A virus. Participants will receive three doses of either vaccine within the first six months of the trial and then will be followed for a total of 20 months through periodic clinic visits and contacts.

The current Herpevac Trial is a follow-up of an earlier vaccine study. Previously, about 2,600 people were immunized with a protein subunit vaccine—that is, a portion of HSV-2 glycoprotein D combined with an **adjuvant**, a substance that helps stimulate immune response. The vaccine was found to be safe and well tolerated by the subjects, and many developed a measurable immune response. The results were disappointing, though, in that as the subjects continued to be monitored, they showed no significant protection from subsequent HSV infection. However, later analyses of specific subgroups within the study revealed that one group was significantly protected. The vaccine was effective in 75% of women who had tested negative for both HSV-1 and HSV-2 infection. For reasons that are not clear, the vaccine was not effective in men or in women who were already infected with HSV-1.

The current Herpevac Trial is designed to produce neutralizing antibody in uninfected women. There is no chance of developing genital herpes from the vaccine, since it contains no infectious virus, only a protein subunit. The glycoprotein D antigen being used in the vaccine is an important protein for virus attachment and entry into host cells. If the immune system can produce antibodies that bind to glycoprotein D on the virus and prevent it from entering cells, infection could be stopped (Figure 8.2).

HUMAN DISEASES FOR WHICH VACCINES ARE AVAILABLE	
DISEASE	PATHOGEN
Anthrax	*Bacillus anthracis*
Whooping cough	*Bordetella pertussis*
Tetanus	*Clostridium tetani*
Diphtheria	*Corynebacterium diphtheria*
Chicken pox	Varicella zoster virus
Smallpox	Variola virus
German measles	Rubella virus

Scientists are hopeful that it is just a matter of time before an effective HSV vaccine is available. The first human herpesvirus vaccine was developed against varicella zoster virus in Japan in 1974. The vaccine consists of a live, attenuated virus that induces protective immunity but does not cause clinical disease. Chicken pox, once a rite of passage of childhood, will no longer be experienced by future generations. The varicella vaccine was investigated extensively in the United States before approval in

HUMAN DISEASES FOR WHICH NO VACCINE EXISTS

DISEASE	PATHOGEN
AIDS	Human immunodeficeny virus (HIV)
Genital herpes	Herpes simplex virus (HSV)
Lyme disease	*Borrelia burgdorferi*
Legionnaires' disease	*Legionella pneumophila*
Gonorrhea	*Neisseria gonorrhoeae*
Syphilis	*Treponema pallidum*
Infant bronchiolitis	Respiratory syncytial virus (RSV)
Dengue fever	Dengue fever virus

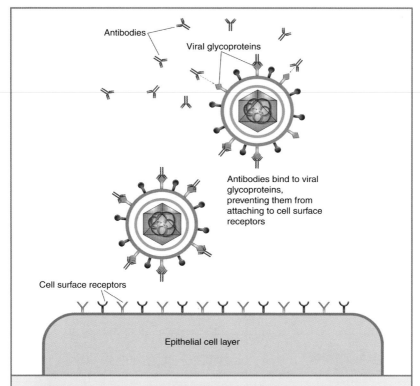

Figure 8.2 Immunization against HSV is designed to develop neutralizing antibodies in people who receive the vaccine. The vaccine contains viral glycoprotein D, an essential factor for virus attachment and entry into host cells. If immunized individuals can produce an immune response to glycoprotein D, the resulting antibodies will bind to the viral glycoprotein and prevent it from binding to host cell surface receptors. This effectively neutralizes the virus and protects those who are vaccinated from virus infection.

1995, and it has now been recommended for routine childhood vaccination and for susceptible older children and adults. Twenty states currently require that children entering public school receive the chicken pox vaccine, and it is expected that many more states will adopt this requirement.

Although the live attenuated vaccine was successful in the case of varicella zoster virus, similar attempts for generating

THE NATIONAL INSTITUTES OF HEALTH

The National Institutes of Health (NIH) dates back to 1887, where it began as a one-room "Laboratory of Hygiene" within the Marine Hospital Service (MHS) on Staten Island, New York. In the 1880s, Congress charged the MHS with the task of screening passengers on arriving ships for signs of infectious disease, such as cholera and yellow fever, with the aim of preventing epidemics. Dr. Joseph Kinyon was the first investigator at the Laboratory of Hygiene, and he set out to identify and search for cures for the infectious diseases that were threatening the lives of American citizens. Intensive research led to the identification of the origin and causes of cholera, diphtheria, typhoid, smallpox, plague, and tuberculosis.

The progress and success of the Laboratory of Hygiene convinced many members of Congress that research could lead to cures for human disease. Congress mandated an expansion and reorganization of the laboratory, which was subsequently renamed the National Institutes of Health. In 1938, the growing research institution moved to its current headquarters in Bethesda, Maryland.

Today, the NIH is the largest single source of funding for biomedical research, with an annual budget near $28 billion. The goal of NIH research is to acquire new knowledge to help prevent, detect, diagnose, and treat disease and disability, from the rarest genetic disorder to the common cold. The mission of the NIH is to uncover new knowledge that will lead to better health for everyone. The NIH, now comprising 27 separate institutes and centers, is one of eight health agencies of the Public Health Service, which, in turn, is part of the U.S. Department of Health and Human Services.

immunity to HSV have not yet been successful. Protein subunit vaccines like Herpevac currently hold the most promise for protecting future generations from genital herpes. In the absence of an effective vaccine against HSV, education is the primary defense against the spread of this virus. Making people aware of the signs and symptoms of genital herpes is of paramount importance for slowing this burgeoning epidemic. Because genital herpes is spread through sexual activity, parents and teachers tend not to discuss the topic openly with teenagers, who represent a significant risk group. Physicians often have more serious and life-threatening issues to deal with when treating patients, and rarely warn them about the dangers of genital herpes.

The Division of STD Prevention at the Centers for Disease Control and Prevention (CDC) recently examined the need for prevention programs for viral STDs other than HIV. An important outcome was the finding that at many clinics, routine STD testing does not include a test for HSV. New standards require that patients be offered type-specific HSV serology testing or be informed if HSV testing is not part of the overall STD evaluation. In addition, the CDC is taking a more aggressive stance toward the prevention of neonatal herpes though serological testing of pregnant women. Finally, initiating a campaign to better educate health-care providers and the general public about genital herpes and promote responsible sexual behavior is also a top priority of the Centers for Disease Control and Prevention's National Center for HIV, STDs, and TB (tuberculosis) Prevention.

9

The Future of Herpes

When Paul Ehrlich first described his "magic bullet" theory in the early 1900s, many scientists were skeptical. Ehrlich's idea was that one could find chemicals to kill specific pathogens while leaving the surrounding host cells unharmed. Over many years, he tested hundreds of compounds, finally succeeding in finding one that killed the syphilis bacterium without harming the host. Paul Ehrlich was awarded the Nobel Prize in 1908, and since that time, scientists have relished the thought that so-called magic bullets would be found for other diseases as well. In the 1980s, monoclonal antibodies were heralded as the next magic bullets, specifically binding to and targeting cancer cells or HIV-infected cells. Today, monoclonal antibody therapeutics are being used regularly to treat diseases like breast cancer and rheumatoid arthritis. Imagine the next step in this process: not just targeting a cell to destroy it, but targeting it with genetic instructions designed to make it normal again.

Gene therapy, the newest version of the magic bullet, is a technique for correcting the defective genes that are responsible for disease development. The most common approach used is to insert a normal gene into a nonspecific location within the genome to replace a nonfunctional gene. The gene is delivered using a carrier molecule called a **vector**. The most common vectors are viruses that have been genetically modified to carry normal human DNA. Since viruses are already quite adept at delivering their own genetic material to host cells, scientists have tried to take advantage of this property by manipulating the viral genome to remove pathogenic genes and insert therapeutic genes (Figure 9.1).

Several types of viruses have been tested as potential vectors for gene therapy, but one of the leading contenders is HSV. Many features of the

A BRIEF HISTORY OF GENE THERAPY

Ashanti de Silva was born with a rare genetic disease called severe combined immune deficiency, or SCID. She lacked a healthy immune system and was vulnerable to virtually any passing germ. Children with this illness usually succumb to overwhelming infections and rarely survive to adulthood. For the first four years of her life, Ashanti led a sheltered existence, remaining in her sterilized home environment and battling illness after illness. On September 14, 1990, scientists attempted to do the unthinkable—recode Ashanti's genetic makeup.

Ashanti's immune deficiency stemmed from the lack of a specific enzyme, adenosine deaminase (ADA), required for development of healthy lymphocytes. To save her life, doctors removed her blood cells, infected them with a retrovirus containing the gene for the normal ADA enzyme, and then returned the cells. The treatment worked, and Ashanti's immune system became fully functional. Although the effects were not as long-lived as the investigators hoped, the first human gene therapy trial was a success. Although she still requires supplemental treatments, Ashanti is alive and well today, thanks to modern medical technology.

Other gene therapy trials were not as successful as this one, and in 1999, gene therapy suffered a major setback with the death of 18-year-old Jesse Gelsinger. Jesse was participating in a gene therapy trial to replace a deficient metabolic enzyme, ornithine transcarboxylase (OTC). He died from multiple organ failure only four days after starting treatment. The Food and Drug Administration (FDA) temporarily halted gene therapy research to examine ways to improve guidelines for patient safety. Research has resumed, and new gene therapy trials for life-threatening conditions are under way, with close monitoring by the FDA. To date, over 400 gene therapy trials involving more than 3,500 patients have been conducted.

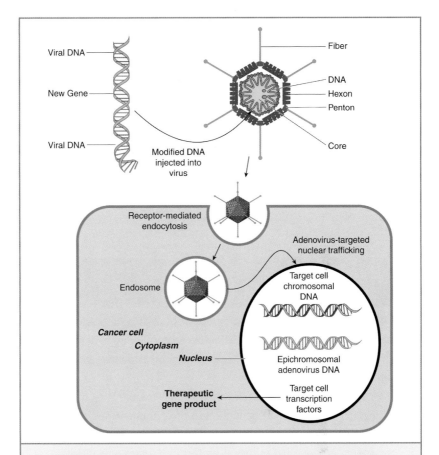

Figure 9.1 Adenovirus-mediated gene therapy involves inserting a human gene into the adenovirus genome. The virus infects the cell, entering the cytoplasm, and then releases the viral DNA into the nucleus. The viral genome, containing the new human gene, is maintained as an extrachromosomal DNA molecule. If the therapy is successful, the host cell will produce the protein encoded by the therapeutic gene and disease symptoms will be alleviated.

virus and its infection cycle make it an attractive candidate for a vector. The viral genome is large and many genes are dispensable for viral function, allowing for insertion of multiple genes. In addition, during latency, HSV is not cleared by the immune system, and the genome remains intact in infected cells for the lifetime of the host without disturbing normal function. Finally, and uniquely among other potential viral vectors, HSV has the ability to infect neurons. A vector capable of delivering genes to nerve cells could be used to kill brain tumors, stimulate regrowth of damaged nerves, treat chronic pain, and protect neurons from further degeneration. Significant effort in this endeavor is already under way in several U.S. research laboratories.

HSV gene therapy vectors may prove useful for the treatment of neurological disorders such as Parkinson's disease.

WHAT OTHER VIRUSES ARE BEING USED FOR GENE THERAPY?

The biggest obstacle to the progress of human gene therapy is the development of safe and effective vectors for gene delivery. In addition to herpes viruses, a number of other delivery vectors are being used.

Retroviruses are a desirable option because they can integrate copies of their genome into the chromosomes of the host cells, allowing for long-lasting therapeutic effects. The downside is that most retroviral vectors can infect only dividing cells, limiting the number of disease targets. Another drawback is that the retroviral genome is inserted into the host DNA; this is good for longevity, but is potentially dangerous if the insertion disrupts another gene with an essential function.

Adenoviruses are another candidate vector that can infect a wide range of cells. Adenoviruses also have large genomes that can accommodate the insertion of large amounts of DNA. They can infect nondividing cells, and they don't insert their genetic material into the genome. The disadvantage of adenoviral vectors is that they are readily cleared by the immune system, often resulting in inflammation and tissue damage.

Parkinson's disease is caused by the selective degeneration of neurons in an area of the brain called the substantia nigra. As these neurons produce less and less of the neurotransmitter dopamine, motor control is affected. Signs of Parkinson's include involuntary tremors, a stooped shuffling gait, and movements that are generally slow and stiff. In animal models of the disease, HSV-vector-based gene therapy studies have successfully reduced degeneration of the dopaminic neurons by delivering a cell survival gene, Bcl-2. Bcl-2 blocks the activation of the apoptosis cascade and promotes cell survival. Continued work in this area aims to develop a system that

Adeno-associated viruses (AAVs) are small viruses that insert their genetic materials into a specific site on chromosome 19. They are useful for gene therapy because long-term expression is possible; they also infect a wide range of cell types, but are less capable of stimulating an immune response than adenoviruses. Unfortunately, AAVs are difficult to produce in high quantities, limiting their usefulness for large-scale studies.

Liposomes are nonviral delivery vectors that consist of an artificial lipid sphere that carries the therapeutic DNA. They deliver the gene by fusing with the target cell membrane and releasing the DNA inside. To date, only low rates of gene delivery have been achieved with this method, and the expression of the gene has been short-lived.

As continued research leads to the development of more efficient delivery methods, gene therapy may be used for the treatment of not only genetic disorders, but also common illnesses like heart disease and cancer.

would be suitable for trials in human Parkinson's disease. Chances for success are promising, given that human trials are beginning for another HSV-vector-based treatment for chronic pain. In this strategy, HSV is being used to deliver **enkephalin** to neurons of the dorsal root ganglion. Enkephalin is a naturally occurring morphine-like substance that acts as an analgesic (pain reliever).

Despite the negative impact HSV can have on the lives of those experiencing severe recurrent outbreaks, there is potential for this virus to improve the quality of life dramatically for many others suffering from debilitating neurological disorders and brain malignancies. In one way or another, the herpes simplex virus will continue to influence humankind for years to come.

Genital Herpes Fact Sheet from the Centers for Disease Control and Prevention

WHAT IS GENITAL HERPES?

Genital herpes is a sexually transmitted disease (STD) caused by the herpes simplex viruses type 1 (HSV-1) and type 2 (HSV-2). Most genital herpes is caused by HSV-2. Most individuals have no or only minimal signs or symptoms from HSV-1 or HSV-2 infection. When signs do occur, they typically appear as one or more blisters on or around the genitals or rectum. The blisters break, leaving tender ulcers (sores) that may take two to four weeks to heal the first time they occur. Typically, another outbreak can appear weeks or months after the first, but it almost always is less severe and shorter than the first outbreak. Although the infection can stay in the body indefinitely, the number of outbreaks tends to decrease over a period of years.

HOW COMMON IS GENITAL HERPES?

Results of a nationally representative study show that genital herpes infection is common in the United States. Nationwide, at least 45 million people ages 12 and older, or one out of five adolescents and adults, have had genital HSV infection. Between the late 1970s and the early 1990s, the number of Americans with genital herpes infection increased 30 percent.

Genital HSV-2 infection is more common in women (approximately one out of four women) than in men (almost one out of five).

This may be due to male-to-female transmissions being more likely than female-to-male transmission.

HOW DO PEOPLE GET GENITAL HERPES?

HSV-1 and HSV-2 can be found in and released from the sores that the viruses cause, but they also are released between outbreaks from skin that does not appear to be broken or to have a sore. Generally, a person can only get HSV-2 infection during sexual contact with someone who has a genital HSV-2 infection. Transmission can occur from an infected partner who does not have a visible sore and may not know that he or she is infected.

HSV-1 can cause genital herpes, but it more commonly causes infections of the mouth and lips, so-called "fever blisters." HSV-1 infection of the genitals can be caused by oral-genital or genital-genital contact with a person who has HSV-1 infection. Genital HSV-1 outbreaks recur less regularly than genital HSV-2 outbreaks.

WHAT ARE THE SIGNS AND
SYMPTOMS OF GENITAL HERPES?

Most people infected with HSV-2 are not aware of their infection. However, if signs and symptoms occur during the first outbreak, they can be quite pronounced. The first outbreak usually occurs within two weeks after the virus is transmitted, and the sores typically heal within two to four weeks. Other signs and symptoms during the primary episode may include a second crop of sores, and flu-like symptoms, including fever and swollen glands. However, most individuals with HSV-2 infection may never have sores, or they may have very mild signs that they do not even notice or that they mistake for insect bites or another skin condition.

Most people diagnosed with a first episode of genital herpes can expect to have several (typically four or five) outbreaks (symptomatic recurrences) within a year. Over time these recurrences usually decrease in frequency.

WHAT ARE THE COMPLICATIONS OF GENITAL HERPES?

Genital herpes can cause recurrent painful genital sores in many adults, and herpes infection can be severe in people with suppressed immune systems. Regardless of severity of symptoms, genital herpes frequently causes psychological distress in people who know they are infected.

In addition, genital HSV can cause potentially fatal infections in babies. It is important that women avoid contracting herpes during pregnancy because a first episode during pregnancy causes a greater risk of transmission to the baby. If a woman has active genital herpes at delivery, a cesarean delivery is usually performed. Fortunately, infection of a baby from a woman with herpes infection is rare.

Herpes may play a role in the spread of HIV, the virus that causes AIDS. Herpes can make people more susceptible to HIV infection, and it can make HIV-infected individuals more infectious.

HOW IS GENITAL HERPES DIAGNOSED?

The signs and symptoms associated with HSV-2 can vary greatly. Health care providers can diagnose genital herpes by visual inspection if the outbreak is typical, and by taking a sample from the sore(s) and testing it in a laboratory. HSV infections can be difficult to diagnose between outbreaks. Blood tests, which detect HSV-1 or HSV-2 infection, may be helpful, although the results are not always clear-cut.

IS THERE A TREATMENT FOR HERPES?

There is no treatment that can cure herpes, but antiviral medications can shorten and prevent outbreaks during the period of time the person takes the medication. In addition, daily suppressive therapy for symptomatic herpes can reduce transmission to partners.

HOW CAN HERPES BE PREVENTED?

The surest way to avoid transmission of sexually transmitted diseases, including genital herpes, is to abstain from sexual contact, or to be in a long-term mutually monogamous relationship with a partner who has been tested and is known to be uninfected.

Genital ulcer diseases can occur in both male and female genital areas that are covered or protected by a latex condom, as well as in areas that are not covered. Correct and consistent use of latex condoms can reduce the risk of genital herpes only when the infected area or site of potential exposure is protected. Since a condom may not cover all infected areas, even correct and consistent use of latex condoms cannot guarantee protection from genital herpes.

Persons with herpes should abstain from sexual activity with uninfected partners when lesions or other symptoms of herpes are present. It is important to know that even if a person does not have any symptoms he or she can still infect sex partners. Sex partners of infected persons should be advised that they may become infected. Sex partners can seek testing to determine if they are infected with HSV. A positive HSV-2 blood test most likely indicates a genital herpes infection.

WHERE CAN I GET MORE INFORMATION?
Division of STD Prevention (DSTDP)
Centers for Disease Control and Prevention
www.cdc.gov/std

Personal health inquiries and information about STDs:
CDC National STD and AIDS Hotlines
(800) 227-8922 or (800) 342-2437
En Espanol (800) 344-7432
TTY for the Deaf and Hard of Hearing (800) 243-7889

National Herpes Hotline
(919) 361-8488

National Herpes Resource Center
http://www.ashastd.org/hrc
herpesnet@ashastd.org

Resources:
CDC National Prevention Information Network (NPIN)
P.O. Box 6003
Rockville, MD 20849-6003
1-800-458-5231
1-888-282-7681 Fax
1-800-243-7012 TTY
www.cdcnpin.org
E-mail: **info@cdcnpin.org**

American Social Health Association (ASHA)
P. O. Box 13827
Research Triangle Park, NC 27709-3827
1-800-783-9877
www.ashastd.org
STD questions: **std-hivnet@ashastd.org**

Epidemiology and Natural History of HSV2
World Health Organization Report, 2001

EPIDEMIOLOGY OF HSV2

HSV2 prevalence is increasing worldwide, . . . and HSV2 is the major cause of genital ulcer disease (GUD) in the developed world. In the developing world, the major public health importance of HSV2 lies in its potential role as a co-factor for HIV transmission.

The high prevalence of HSV2 in many populations results from the fact that it is a lifelong infection, which is highly infectious and often transmitted in the absence of symptoms. There have been few data on HSV2 prevalence until recent years, when type-specific serology became available, enabling researchers to estimate HSV prevalence and incidence. However, there is currently concern about the specificity of some of these serological assays when used to analyse sera from African countries. . . .

GLOBAL EPIDEMIOLOGY OF HSV2

HSV2 prevalence varies widely, with generally higher rates in developing than in developed countries and in urban than in rural areas. Prevalence is higher in the USA (22% in adults) compared with Europe (generally less than 15%). However, substantially higher rates are seen in Sub-Saharan Africa and the Caribbean, with prevalences in adults of around 50% in many countries (Table 1). Overall, prevalence is higher in women compared with men, especially among the young, and rates of up to 40% have been recorded among women aged 15–19 in Kisumu, Kenya. Infection has been associated with younger age at first sex, increased years of sexual activity, increasing number of lifetime partners, lack of circumcision (in men), and current or recent other STIs.

HSV2 AS A MARKER FOR SEXUAL BEHAVIOUR

As HSV2 is more readily transmitted sexually than HIV, HSV2 serology may be a useful marker for changes in sexual behaviour in HIV intervention studies. However, the persistent nature of the infection implies that seroprevalence may not be a sensitive marker of behaviour change, although it will be more discriminating at the lower prevalences seen in younger age groups. HSV2 seroincidence would be a preferable marker of behaviour change, especially in countries in sub-Saharan Africa where there is high incidence among young people.

IDENTIFIED GAPS IN KNOWLEDGE

There are currently few data on HSV2 prevalence from many parts of the world, including Asia, South America and many parts of Africa. HSV2 incidence data are also scarce. Prevalence and incidence data are necessary: i) to estimate population attributable fractions (PAFs) for HIV; ii) as background data to inform future intervention studies, such as HSV2 treatment and vaccine trials; iii) to evaluate the need for changes in syndromic management of GUD due to presence of genital herpes; and iv) to evaluate the need for regular HSV2 seroprevalence surveys.

Genital herpes can also be due to HSV1 infection, and a study in Scotland found that 40% of genital herpes was due to HSV1 in 1991. Both HSV1 and HSV2 are able to infect and reactivate in the same anatomic area, although the natural history of these infections is markedly different, with HSV2 recurring more frequently than HSV1, so most clinical reactivations are likely to be due to HSV2. In developing countries, the proportion of genital herpes caused by HSV1 is unknown, although assumed to be low.

Among HIV-negative pregnant women living in developed countries, the risk of neonatal herpes is very low.

Table 1 HSV2 Seroprevalence in General Population in Developing Countries

COUNTRY	POPULATION	YEAR	PREVALENCE[1]
Uganda	Adults (rural)	1989	74% (f); 57% (m)
Congo	Adults (urban)	1982	0.71
Kenya	Adults (urban)	1997	68% (f); 35% (m)
Zambia	Adults (urban)	1997	55% (f); 36% (m)
Rwanda	Hospital Workers (rural)	1985	0.51
Cameroon	Adults (urban)	1997	51% (f); 27% (m)
Costa Rica	Adult women	1985	43% (f)
Tanzania	Adults (rural)	1993	42% (f); 19% (m)[2]
Brazil	Adults (urban)	1990/91	0.42
Zaire	Adults (urban)	1985	0.41
Rwanda	Adults (rural)	1985	0.33
Benin	Adults (urban)	1997	30% (f); 12% (m)
Brazil	Blood donors (urban)	1994	0.29
Rwanda	Army Recruits (rural)	1985	28% (m)
Senegal	Surgical patients (urban)	1985	0.2
Philippines	Adults (urban)	1991/93	0.09
China	Gynaecology clinic (urban)	1984/85	2% (f)

[1] (f) females; (m) males
[2] Age-weighted sample: younger age-groups were over-represented

RECOMMENDATIONS
Analysis of sera from past and present studies for HSV2 prevalence

HSV2 testing of stored sera from existing cohorts was recommended as a source of additional data to understand past as well as current prevalence and trends. However, there are currently problems with specificity of serological tests on African sera.

Use of sentinel surveillance sera to obtain HSV2 prevalence data in different populations, especially in Asia and South America

Analysis of sera collected through routine sentinel surveillance would allow estimation of HSV2 prevalence in populations in which few data are available. Suitable sentinel populations may follow the HIV surveillance model: in areas of low prevalence, the focus would be on core groups, whereas in areas of high prevalence, data for the general population would be more relevant. Antenatal clinic (ANC) surveillance systems established to monitor HIV could also be used to record HSV2 prevalence. Possible sources of bias in using ANC data to represent the general population may differ from those reported for HIV.

Consideration could be given to the routine inclusion of HSV2 serology in established sentinel surveillance systems, particularly in populations where HSV2 is thought to account for a substantial proportion of HIV infections.

Estimation of seroprevalence should include young age-groups. As they are more sensitive to changes in behaviour patterns than are older age groups, such data should be more informative of the current situation.

Estimating the proportion of genital herpes caused by HSV1 in developing countries

Little is known about the proportion of genital herpes caused by HSV1 in developing countries. Aetiological studies of ulcers performed in areas of high HIV prevalence should also include specific HSV1 testing.

Estimating the burden of neonatal herpes in developing countries

Anecdotal reports suggest that neonatal herpes is rarely seen in Africa. However, the frequency of this outcome may be increased in areas of high HIV prevalence because of the increased risk of HSV2 genital shedding in HIV infected women.

An indication of the potential for vertical transmission of HSV2 could be obtained by measuring HSV2 incidence during pregnancy in existing studies, e.g.:

- the Rakai sub-study on pregnant women

- seroincidence studies in pregnant women participating in programmes to prevent perinatal transmission of HIV.

Natural History of HSV2

CLINICAL COURSE OF HSV2 INFECTION

The clinical spectrum of HSV2 includes primary infection with the virus (either HSV1 or HSV2), the first clinical episode of genital herpes, and recurrent episodes of clinical disease. The median recurrence rate after a symptomatic first episode of genital herpes is four to five episodes per year, and severe first episodes are associated with even higher recurrence rates. In addition, subclinical or "asymptomatic" infection may be associated with infectious viral shedding. The proportion of infections that are both symptomatic and recognized (by patient and clinician) is estimated to vary between 13% and 37%, although this is higher among HIV-positive individuals. This proportion may increase with provision of health education regarding signs and symptoms of herpes. For example, 50–75% of HSV2 seropositive subjects without a history of genital herpes have reported subsequent symptomatic episodes after receiving health education on genital herpes.

The natural history of herpes infection is poorly documented in low-income countries, and, to our knowledge, no long-term prospective studies of HSV2 shedding have been carried out in developing countries.

TRANSMISSION AND ACQUISITION OF HSV2 INFECTION

The amount of shedding required for HSV2 transmission to occur is unknown. In a prospective study of HSV2-discordant partners, most transmission events were not associated with a clinically recognized HSV2 recurrence in the infected partner. As for other STIs, the risk of acquisition of HSV2 seems to be higher in women than in men. This may relate to the higher number of HSV2 recurrences in infected men (about 20% higher than in women), to biological factors such as the larger and more vulnerable mucosal surface of women, or possibly to differences in awareness and reporting of symptoms between women and men.

INTERACTION BETWEEN HSV1 AND HSV2

In developed countries, acquisition of HSV1 in childhood has decreased as HSV2 seroprevalence has increased, suggesting a possible protective effect of HSV1 against HSV2 acquisition. However, studies have shown discrepant results in this respect. Although HSV1 does not seem to modify the risk of HSV2 acquisition, it seems to increase the proportion of asymptomatic seroconversions and, in one study, to increase the rate of HSV2 shedding. Infection with HSV1 in childhood is almost universal in many developing countries, where HSV2 prevalence is also very high, and this confirms that HSV1 provides limited protection against infection with HSV2.

Appendix II

RECOMMENDATIONS
Studies on the natural history of HSV2 nested within intervention studies

More information is needed on the natural history of HSV2 in developing countries. Such studies could be nested within HIV intervention studies, and could examine the effect of HIV infection on natural history of HSV2. These studies should be conducted in countries with high rates of HIV and HSV2 infection. The prospective nature of intervention studies will allow: i) estimation of the duration of primary infection, which determines frequency of shedding and recurrence rates; ii) assessment of differences in recurrence and shedding according to HIV and circumcision status; and iii) assessment of the effects of other factors, such as nutritional status and poor hygiene.

There are several issues to consider in the design of such cohort studies: i) the need to include young age-groups, not yet sexually active, in order to obtain data on primary infection; ii) losses to follow-up; iii) ethical issues, such as provision of voluntary counselling and testing services for HIV, antiretroviral therapy and aciclovir for severe herpetic episodes; iv) identification of cases will require regular serological surveys (probably six-monthly); v) the overall duration of follow-up required is unclear; vi) such studies should be performed in a site allowing good clinical follow-up.

Use of existing data from trials and cohort studies to estimate HSV2 transmission rates and to identify factors affecting transmission

More data are needed on transmission rates of HSV2 and factors influencing transmission. There is an urgent need to analyse existing data generated in studies performed by different research groups. Current data may help to address the problem of unrecognized infection and subclinical viral shedding, which appear to be major factors in transmission. Transmission should be examined according to stage of infection, symptom status, sex, HIV status and condom use.

New studies to examine HSV2 transmission

Two types of study were recommended to examine HSV2 transmission: studies designed to identify and interview partners of patients with newly-diagnosed genital herpes and studies of discordant couples for HSV2. In both cases careful consideration should be given to appropriate counselling and treatment.

Glossary

Adjuvant—A substance that enhances the effectiveness of a medical treatment, such as a vaccine.

Anterograde transport—Movement of material from the cell body of a neuron into the axon.

Apoptosis—Regulated process leading to cell death.

Asymptomatic—Not characterized by obvious clinical signs or symptoms.

Attenuated—Weakened or nonpathogenic, as in bacterial or viral strains used for vaccines.

Beta-lactamase—An enzyme that cleaves the beta-lactam ring of penicillin, rendering the drug ineffective at inhibiting bacterial growth.

Capsid—The protein shell that houses the genetic material of a virus.

Central dogma of biology—Fundamental concept of molecular biology that states that genetic information is stored in the form of DNA, transcribed to a working copy of RNA, and then translated into proteins that perform cellular functions.

Eczema herpeticum—A severe HSV infection that affects the skin, causing chicken pox–like blisters.

Electron microscope—A device that uses an electron beam to produce high magnification, high resolution images.

Endoplasmic reticulum—Part of the cell's cytomembrane system, a double-layered membrane that folds back on itself, creating a series of tubes and layered sacs; functions as the site of synthesis for secreted and membrane proteins.

Enkephalin—Morphine-like neuropeptide produced in the nervous system.

Enzyme—Proteins that increase the rate of biochemical reactions, such as the replication of DNA.

Epidemiology—The study of the factors that determine the frequency and distribution of disease, injury, or other health-related events and their cause in defined human populations.

Episome—A stable, circular piece of DNA maintained in the nucleus separately from the cell's chromosomes.

Gene therapy—The introduction of genetic material into the body to replace faulty or missing genetic material, thus treating or curing a disease or abnormal medical condition.

Genital herpes—An incurable sexually transmitted disease in which painful blisters may appear on the vagina, labia, inner thighs, penis, or anus.

Genome—The totality of an organism's genetic information.

Gingivostomatitis—Disease in which sores appear on the mouth and gums.

Glycoprotein spikes—Proteins that contain carbohydrate moieties and extend from a membrane.

Herpes encephalitis—An acute HSV infection that causes inflammation of the brain and can lead to death.

Herpes gladiatorum—An HSV infection that causes lesions on skin surfaces, particularly on the chest.

Herpes simplex virus (HSV)—A DNA virus that infects human epithelial cells, causing a range of localized skin lesions or other clinical manifestations.

Herpetic keratitis—An HSV infection that affects the eye and can cause vision loss.

Herpetic whitlow—A painful HSV infection of the hand.

HSV meningitis—A complication of genital herpes in which the meninges (membranes surrounding the brain and spinal cord) become inflamed.

Latency—A period of infection in which viral DNA may be present but no infectious virus particles are being produced.

Microscopy—The use of light or electrons to view extremely small objects.

Morphology—Structure or shape.

Mucous membranes—Epithelial cell surfaces covering the body's interior surfaces and the eye.

Necrosis—Cell death resulting from tissue damage.

Neurotropic—Targeting cells of the nervous system.

Nuclear pore—Opening in the nuclear membrane containing proteins that regulate traffic of materials into and out of the nucleus.

Nucleocapsid—A viral capsid containing the viral genome.

Oral herpes—Cold sores, fever blisters, or lesions in the facial region or mouth, usually caused by herpes simplex virus type 1.

Pathogen—A disease-causing microorganism, such as a bacterium, virus, or fungus.

Perinatal—Occurring just before, during, or after birth.

Pharyngitis—Inflammation of the throat.

Plasmid—Small, usually circular DNA molecule found in some bacteria that encode nonvital functions.

Glossary

Polymerase—An enzyme that joins together subunits to form a macro-molecule.

Primary infection—The first exposure to virus resulting in virus replication and often disease in the human host. Following the primary infection, herpes viruses establish latency and the patient may later suffer from recurrent infection.

Prodromal—Mild symptoms occurring prior to the onset of disease.

Proteoglycans—Molecules consisting of one or more glycosaminoglycans chains attached to a core protein.

Retrograde axonal transport—Movement of materials from the axon of a neuron to the cell body.

Retrovirus—Type of virus that converts its RNA genome to DNA by reverse transcriptase as part of its life cycle.

Rolling circle replication—Method used by viruses and some bacteria to copy circular DNA genomes. The circular DNA is nicked on one strand, which is then used as a template to make more copies of the genome in a very rapid manner, resulting in a long tail of newly replicated genomes trailing off the original circular genome.

Scaffolding proteins—Proteins that provide structural support during assembly.

Sexually transmitted disease (**STD**)—Any disease that is contracted through sexual intercourse or intimate sexual contact. STDs include syphilis, gonorrhea, chlamydia, and genital herpes.

Tegument—Dense protein layer located between the capsid and envelope of herpes viruses.

Transcription—Copying one strand of DNA into a complementary RNA sequence.

Translation—Process by which the sequence of nucleotides encoded in an mRNA molecule directs the incorporation of amino acids into a protein.

Vaccine—An agent that confers immunity without causing disease.

Vector—An agent used for transmission of a pathogen or genetic material.

Virion—An intact, nonreplicating virus particle.

Virologist—A scientist who studies viruses.

Virology—The study of viruses and diseases caused by viruses.

Virus—A microscopic packet of nucleic acid wrapped in a protein coat.

Adachi, N., D. L. Konu, K. Frei, et al. "The HSV-TK/GCV Gene Therapy for Brain Tumors." *Gene Therapy and Molecular Biology* 4 (1999): 248–260.

Arbeter, A. M., S. E. Starr, and S. A. Plotkin. "Varicella Vaccine Studies in Healthy Children and Adults." *Pediatrics* 78(1986): 748–756.

Arvin, A. M., and C. G. Prober. "Herpes Simplex Virus Type 2—A Persistent Problem" (Editorial). *New England Journal of Medicine* 337(1997): 1158–1159.

Bearer, E. L., X. O. Breakefield, D. Schuback, et al. "Retrograde Axonal Transport of Herpes Simplex Virus: Evidence for a Single Mechanism and a Role for Tegument." *Proceedings of the National Academy of Sciences* 97(2000): 8146–8150.

Brener, N., R. Lowry, L. Kann, et al. "Trends in Sexual Risk Behaviors Among High School Students—United States, 1991–2001." *Morbidity and Mortality Weekly Report* 51(2002): 856–859.

Burton, E. A., J. B. Wechuck, S. K. Wendell, et al. "Multiple Applications For Replication-Defective Herpes Simplex Virus Vectors." *Stem Cells* 19(2001): 358–377.

Celum, C. L. "The Interaction Between Herpes Simplex Virus And Human Immunodeficiency Virus." *Herpes* 11, Supplement 1(2004): 36A–45A.

Cohrs, R. J., and D. H. Gilden. "Human Herpesvirus Latency." *Brain Pathology* 11(2001): 465–474.

Dolan, A., F. E. Jamieson, C. Cunningham, et al. "The Genome Sequence of Herpes Simplex Virus Type 2." *Journal of Virology* 72(1998): 2010–2021.

Douglas, M. W., R. J. Diefenbach, F. L. Homa, et al. "Herpes Simplex Virus Type 1 Capsid Protein VP26 Interacts With Dynein Light Chains RP3 and Tctex1 and Plays a Role in Retrograde Cellular Transport." *Journal of Biological Chemistry* 279(2004): 28522–28530.

Fields, B. N., D. M. Knipe, and P. M. Howley, eds. *Fields Virology*, 3rd ed. Philadelphia: Lippincott-Raven Publishers, 1996.

Fleming, D. T., G. M. McQuillan, R. E. Johnson, et al. "Herpes Simplex Virus Type 2 in the United States, 1976–1994." *New England Journal of Medicine* 337(1997): 1105–1111.

Gottlieb, S., J. M. Douglas, Jr., M. Foster, et al. "Incidence of Herpes Simplex Virus Type 2 Infection in 5 Sexually Transmitted Disease (STD) Clinics

Bibliography

and the Effect of HIV/STD Risk-Reduction Counseling." *Journal of Infectious Diseases* 190(2004): 1059–1067.

Greenwood, D., R.C.B. Slack, and J. F. Peutherer. *Medical Microbiology,* 16th ed. Edinburgh, Scotland: Churchill Livingstone, 2002.

Gupta, R., A. Wald, E. Krantz, S. Selke, et al. "Valacyclovir and Acyclovir for Suppression of Shedding of Herpes Simplex Virus in the Genital Tract." *Journal of Infectious Diseases* 190(2004): 1374–1381.

Halioua, B., and J. E. Malkin. "Epidemiology of Genital Herpes—Recent Advances." *European Journal of Dermatology* 9(1999): 177–184.

"How Does Herpes Simplex Type 2 Influence Human Immunodefiency Virus Infection and Pathogenesis?" (editorial) *Journal of Infectious Diseases* 187(2003): 1509–1512.

Hui, E.K., and S. J. Lo. "Does the Latency-Associated Transcript (LAT) of Herpes Simplex Virus Function as a Ribozyme During Viral Reactivation?" *Virus Genes* 16(1998): 147–148.

Ingraham, J. L., and C. A. Ingraham. *Introduction to Microbiology,* 3rd ed. Pacific Grove, CA: Brooks/Cole-Thomson Learning, Inc., 2004.

Koelle, D. M., and L. Corey. "Recent Progress in Herpes Simplex Virus Immunobiology and Vaccine Research." *Clinical Microbiology Reviews* 16(2003): 96–113.

Lodish, H., et al. *Molecular Biology of the Cell,* 5th ed. New York: W. H. Freeman and Co., 2004.

Mahon, C. R., and G. Manuselis, eds. *Textbook of Diagnostic Microbiology.* Philadelphia: W. B. Saunders Company, 2000.

Murray, P., K. S. Rosenthal, G. S. Kobayashi, and M. A. Phaller. *Medical Microbiology.* St. Louis: Mosby, Inc., 2002.

Newcomb, W. W., F. L. Homa, D. R. Thomsen, et al. "Assembly of the Herpes Simplex Virus Procapsid From Purified Components and Identification of Small Complexes Containing the Major Capsid and Scaffolding Proteins." *Journal of Virology* 73(1999): 4239–4250.

Palmer, J. A., R. H. Branston, C. E. Lilley, et al. "Development and Optimization of Herpes Simplex Virus Vectors for Multiple Long-Term Gene Delivery to the Peripheral Nervous System." *Journal of Virology* 74(2000): 5604–5618.

Renzi, C., J. M. Douglas, M. Foster, et al. "Herpes Simplex Virus Type 2 Infection as a Risk Factor for Human Immunodefiency Virus Acquisition in Men Who Have Sex With Men." *Journal of Infectious Diseases* 187(2003): 19–25.

Reynolds, S. J., A. R. Risbund, M. E. Shepard, et al. "Recent Herpes Simplex Type 2 Infection and the Risk of Human Immunodeficiency Virus Type 1 Acquisition in India." *Journal of Infectious Diseases* 187(2003): 1513–1521.

Sheaffer, A. K., W. W. Newcomb, J. C. Brown, et al. "Evidence for the Controlled Incorporation of the Herpes Simplex Virus Type-1 UL26 Protease into Capsids." *Journal of Virology* 74(2000): 6838–6844.

Spear, P. G. "Herpes Simplex Virus: Receptors and Ligands for Cell Entry." *Cellular Microbiology* 6(2004): 401–410.

Spencer, J. V. "Structure and Assembly of the Herpes Simplex Virus Capsid." Ph.D. dissertation, University of Virginia, 1998.

Spencer, J. V., W. W. Newcomb, D. R. Thomsen, et al. "Assembly of the Herpes Simplex Virus Capsid: Preformed Triplexes Bind to the Nascent Capsid." *Journal of Virology* 72(1998): 3944–3951.

Spriggs, M. "One Step Ahead Of the Game: Viral Immunomodulatory Molecules." *Annual Review of Immunology* 14(1996): 101–130.

Stanberry, L. R., S. L. Spruance, A. L. Cunningham, et al. "Glycoprotein D— Adjuvant Vaccine to Prevent Genital Herpes." *New England Journal of Medicine* 347(2002): 1652–1661.

Voyles, B. A. *The Biology of Viruses.* New York: McGraw-Hill, 2002.

Wagner, E. K., and M. J. Hewlett. *Basic Virology*, 2nd ed. Malden, MA: Blackwell Science Ltd., 2004.

Yamada, M., T. Olingino, M. Mata, et al. "Herpes Simplex Virus Vector-Mediated Expression of Bcl-2 Prevents 6-Hydroxydopamine-Induced Degeneration of Neurons in the Substantia Nigra In Vivo." *Proceedings of the National Academy of Sciences* 96(1999): 4078–4083.

Yewdell, J. W., and J. R. Bennink. "Mechanisms of Viral Interference with MHC Class I Antigen Processing and Presentation." *Annual Review of Cell and Developmental Biology* 15(1999): 579–606.

Further Reading

Cunningham, A. H. *Clinician's Manual on Genital Herpes.* Newbury, Berkshire, UK.: LibraPharm Ltd., 1999.

Ebel, Charles, and Anna Wald. *Managing Herpes: How to Live and Love with a Chronic STD.* Research Triangle Park, NC: American Social Health Association, 1994.

Handsfield, H. Hunter. *Genital Herpes.* New York: McGraw-Hill, 2001.

Monif, Gilles. *Understanding Genital Herpes: To Conquer a Dragon (Women's Health Care Series),* 2nd ed. Omaha: IDI Publishers, 1994.

Parker, James, and Philip Parker, eds. *The Official Patient's Sourcebook on Genital Herpes: A Revised and Updated Directory for the Internet Age.* San Diego: Icon Health Publications, 2002.

Sacks, Stephen. *The Truth About Herpes.* West Vancouver, B.C., Canada: Gordon Soules Book Publishers, Ltd., 1997.

Stanberry, Lawrence R. *Understanding Herpes (Understanding Health and Sickness Series).* Jackson, MS: University Press of Mississippi, 1998.

Websites

All the Virology on the World Wide Web—Herpesviruses
http://www.virology.net/garryfavweb12.html#Herpe

American Social Health Association,
National Herpes Resource Center
http://www.ashastd.org/hrc/educate.html

The Buckminster Fuller Institute
http://www.bfi.org

Centers for Disease Control and Prevention,
Division of Sexually Transmitted Diseases: Genital Herpes
http://www.cdc.gov/nchstp/dstd/HerpesInfo.htm

Ernst Ruska: The Nobel Prize in Physics 1986
http://nobelprize.org/physics/laureates/1986

Gertrude Elion: The Nobel Prize in Physiology or Medicine 1988
http://nobelprize.org/medicine/laureates/1988/index.html

Herpevac Trial for Women
http://www.niaid.nih.gov/dmid/stds/herpevac

Medline Plus: Herpes Simplex
http://www.nlm.nih.gov/medlineplus/herpessimplex.html

National Institutes of Health Herpes Fact Sheet
http://www.niaid.nih.gov/factsheets/stdherp.htm

Index

Index

Primary infection, 13, 108
Procapsid, 38
Prodromal (defined), 108
Prodromal symptoms, 64
Proteoglycans, 44, 108
Provirus, 23

Reactivation, 16, 27, 61–62
Replication
of DNA, 32–33, 48–49
of viral genome, 50
of viruses. *See* Virus replication
Retrograde axonal transport, 58, 108
Retrovirus, 23, 30, 90, 108
Reverse transcriptase, 23
Rhabdovirus, 34
RNA, 30
Rolling circle replication, 48, 51, 108
Ruska, Ernst, 36

Salk, Jonas, 79, 80
Scaffolding proteins, 35, 38, 108
SCID (severe combined immune deficiency), 88
Sensory neurons, 55
Serology, 74

Severe combined immune deficiency (SCID), 88
Sexually transmitted disease (STD). *See also specific diseases*
coinfections, 69, 95, 99
defined, 17, 108
incidence, 10, 17, 19
and infertility, 71
list of, 18
prevention and control, 25–27, 86
tests for, 73–74, 86
transmission, 17, 19–21
Sexual partners, multiple, 25–26
Shingles, 10
Skin infections, 65–67
STD. *See* Sexually transmitted disease
Suppressive therapy, 78
Syphilis, 18

Tegument, 15, 38, 108
Tests for STDs, 73–74, 86
Thymidine kinase, 76
Topical treatments, 78
Transcription, 30, 108
Translation, 30, 108
Treatments, 74–75, 78, 95

Trigeminal ganglion, 57

Vaccines
defined, 108
HSV-2, 81–83
poliovirus, 79–81
varicella zoster virus, 83–84
Valtrex (valacyclovir), 74
van Leeuwenhoek, Antoni, 35
Varicella zoster virus, 10, 11, 78, 83–84
Vectors, 87, 108. *See also* Gene therapy
Venereal diseases. *See* Sexually transmitted diseases
Viral culture, 73–74
Virion, 33, 108
Virologist, 15, 108
Virology, 14, 108
Viruses, 108
discovery, 13–14
as gene therapy vectors, 87–92
Virus latency. *See* Latency
Virus replication, 42–53
assembly, 50
attachment and entry, 44–45
DNA replication, 32–33, 48–50
expression, 46–47
genome uncoating, 45–46
release, 50, 52–53

Index

Picture Credits

9: © Dr. Gopal Murti/Visuals Unlimited
12: © Mediscan/Visuals Unlimited
15: © Peter Lamb
20: Library of Congress, LC-USZC2-1119
24: © Peter Lamb
26: © Peter Lamb
29: Courtesy the Public Health Image Library (PHIL), CDC
31: © Peter Lamb
34: © Peter Lamb
37: © Peter Lamb
40: Associated Press, AP/Jim Palmer
43: © Peter Lamb
45: © Dr. Dennis Kunkel/Visuals Unlimited
47: © Dr. K. G. Murti/Visuals Unlimited
49: © Peter Lamb
51: © Peter Lamb

52: © George Musil/Visuals Unlimited
53: © Peter Lamb
56: © Lester V. Bergman/CORBIS
57: © Peter Lamb
59: © Peter Lamb
62: © Peter Lamb
64: © Mediscan/Visuals Unlimited
65: © Dr. Charles J. Ball/CORBIS
66: © Ken Greer/Visuals Unlimited
72: Courtesy CDC
73: © Biodisc/Visuals Unlimited
75: © Peter Lamb
77: Associated Press, AP/Karen Tam
80: (top) Associated Press, AP
80: (bottom) Courtesy PHIL, CDC
84: © Peter Lamb
89: © Peter Lamb

Cover: © Dr. F.A. Murphy/Visuals Unlimited

About the Author

Juliet V. Spencer, Ph.D., is a professor of biology at the University of San Francisco in San Francisco, California. She received her doctoral training at the University of Virginia, studying the structure and assembly of HSV-1 capsid particles, and then performed post-doctoral research on the immune response to influenza virus infection. Dr. Spencer came to USF from the biotechnology industry, where she worked on the development of therapeutics for ovarian cancer and inflammatory diseases. Her current research interests include virus-host interactions and modulation of immune cell function by human herpes viruses.

About the Editor

The late I. Edward Alcamo was a Distinguished Teaching Professor of Microbiology at the State University of New York at Farmingdale. Alcamo studied biology at Iona College in New York and earned his M.S. and Ph.D. degrees in microbiology at St. John's University, also in New York. He had taught at Farmingdale for over 30 years. In 2000, Alcamo won the Carski Award for Distinguished Teaching in Microbiology, the highest honor for microbiology teachers in the United States. He was a member of the American Society for Microbiology, the National Association of Biology Teachers, and the American Medical Writers Association. Alcamo authored numerous books on the subjects of microbiology, AIDS, and DNA technology as well as the award-winning textbook *Fundamentals of Microbiology*, now in its sixth edition.